CLEAN EATING FOR TWO

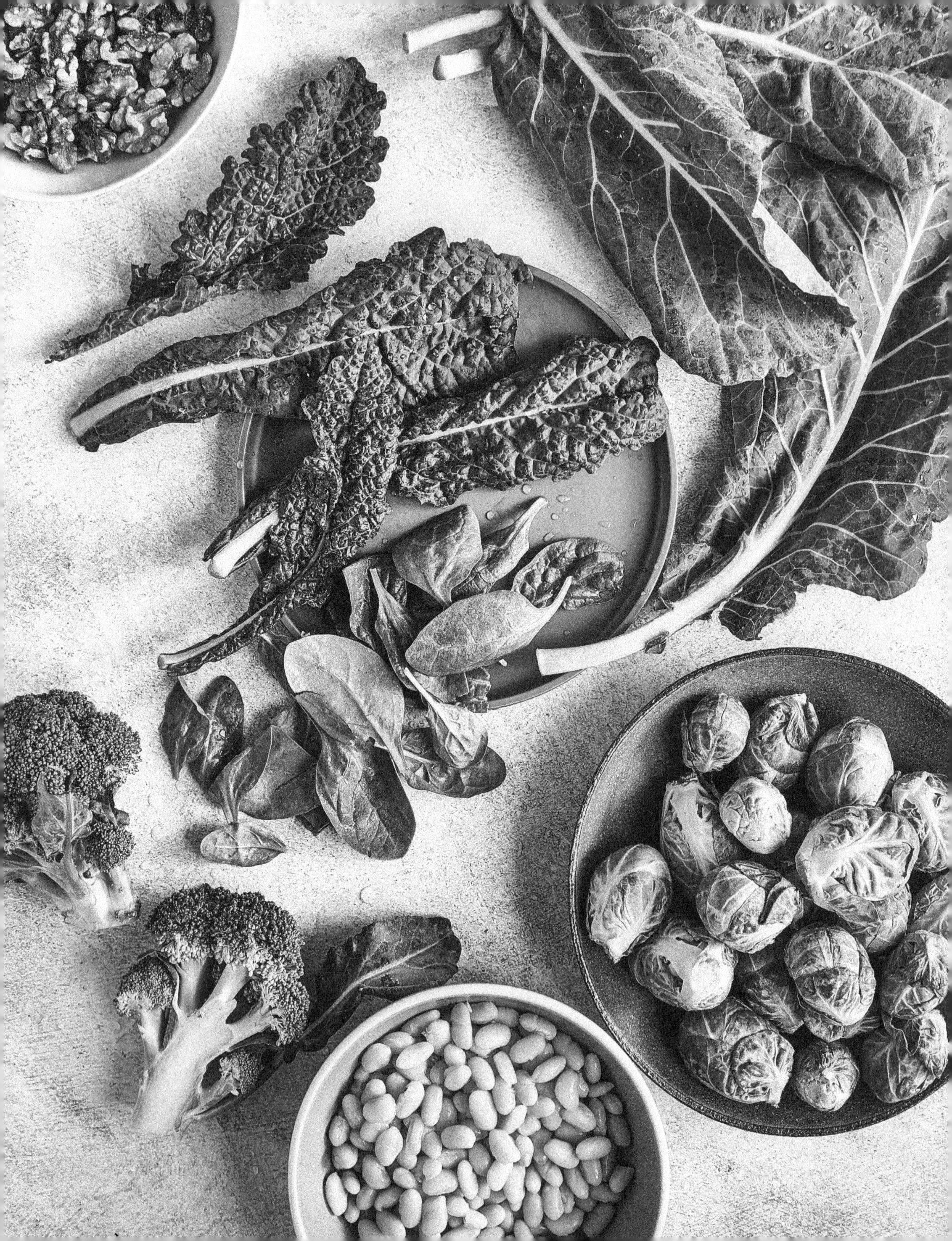

CLEAN EATING FOR TWO

Easy, Fresh Recipes to Eat Healthier Together

MARY OPFER, MS, RD

Photography by Hélène Dujardin

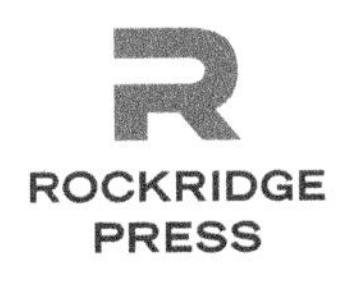

Eddie, Caite, Brian for always supporting me.
Mom, for teaching me how to eat.

Interior and Cover Designer: Mando Daniel
Art Producer: Tom Hood
Editor: Kelly Koester
Production Editor: Rachel Taenzler
Production Manager: Jose Olivera

ISBN: Print 978-1-63807-936-1
eBook 978-1-63807-136-5

R0

CONTENTS

INTRODUCTION

Food brings great pleasure, interest, and comfort to my life. I have worked in the food industry for more than 25 years and have even owned my own restaurant. I took my passion for food and culinary skills, combined them with the science of nutrition, and became a registered dietitian nutritionist, also referred to as an RDN. Currently, I teach graduate-level culinary nutrition courses in which my students and I cook dishes from around the globe and discuss how culture, tradition, and local ingredients make unique cuisines. Along with my experience, I bring my wealth of food knowledge, cooking skills, and passion for food to the recipes and guidance in this book.

My mother was the first to inspire my love for clean eating. Even with seven children, she always put a freshly prepared, nutritious meal on the table three times a day. As kids, my siblings and I were allowed junk food and soft drinks only at birthday parties and on special occasions. I always felt that I was missing out, but today, with lifelong good health and the skills to feed my own family healthily, I realize that I have gained much more than I lost.

After college, I not only began cooking regularly but also fell in love with cooking itself. I realized that perhaps more important than cooking with quality ingredients is cooking with love. Science has yet to pinpoint what makes a home-cooked meal special or what makes grandma's apple pie better than any other. But we know that there is something about the dynamics of cooking with love, purpose, and pride that makes food taste, well, just so much better.

Like most people, I have a busy life. As a full-time professor with two children who for years were involved in many activities, I tried, sometimes in vain, to have family meals. Today, as an empty nester, my husband and I have mastered this. Making time for one another has strengthened our bond and renewed our joy of being together.

A challenge for those cooking for two (including me) is buying only what you need for meals and not much more. Another challenge is making proper portions for two people. I've learned some tips and tricks to help you, and I've included them in this book. For those of you cooking for one, most of the tips will apply. In some cases, you may have a portion left that you can freeze or use for leftovers the next day.

I wrote this cookbook to be a valuable tool in both your kitchen and the supermarket. The first chapter will provide background on the value of clean eating for overall health as well as for weight loss and the prevention and management of various health conditions. Following that are 85 clean-eating recipes that use simple, wholesome, and healthy ingredients.

Think of clean eating as going "back to basics." My recipes do not require hours of prep and cooking or specialty ingredients. All the recipes are created for ease in locating ingredients and preparing the freshest, tastiest dishes in the least amount of time. They are labeled easy in one or more of three ways: one pot, dish, or skillet; five-ingredient (excluding oil/cooking spray, water, and salt and pepper); and quick (30 minutes or less).

The recipes in this book will better your health, bringjoy to you and your partner, help you avoid leftovers or waste, and even help turn clean eating into a new lifestyle.

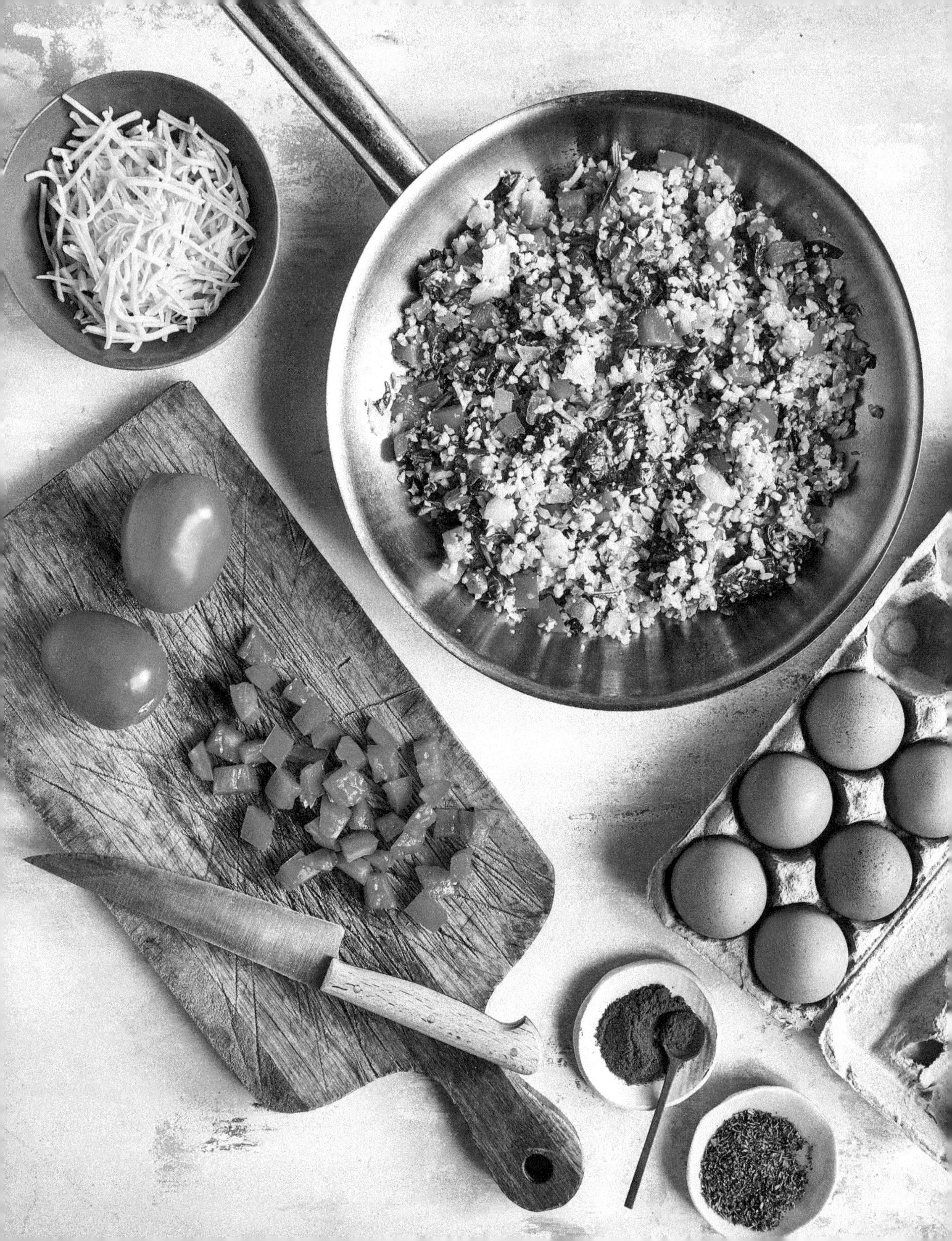

CHAPTER ONE

Eat Clean and Get Healthy Together

So long, processed foods; hello, fresh ingredients. Don't let cooking for two get in the way—this chapter will prepare you to cook meals at home, enjoy nutrient-dense foods, and not be wasteful. I use many of the same ingredients in multiple recipes, making it easy for you to use leftover portions of ingredients like beans, greens, and meat products. Cooking, shopping, and prepping together builds relationships and improves overall health.

What Is Clean Eating?

Welcome to the world of clean eating! If you are looking to make a change to better your health, you are in the right place to start (or continue) your journey. This book will provide you with guidance and tips for preparing quick, simple recipes following the clean-eating fundamentals.

Life is busy, so sometimes healthy eating ends up on the back burner. Tweaking your choices to incorporate more whole foods will help you reach your weight loss or maintenance goals, improve your overall health, and prevent or manage particular health conditions. You don't have to spend hours in the kitchen or loads of money in order to eat healthily and deliciously.

What I love about clean eating is that you are eating real food. It is not a fad or restrictive diet that requires special foods or limits what you can eat. It's adaptable to fit your lifestyle and schedule. A clean-eating diet boosts energy, strengthens immunity, and supports your mood as well as protecting against heart disease, diabetes, and cancer.

Clean eating means prioritizing whole, minimally processed foods such as fruits, vegetables, lean proteins, complex carbs, and healthy fats. Processed foods are those altered from their natural state and typically contain a long list of synthetic ingredients and added sugars—and often with those, lower nutritional value. Of note, clean eating does not exclude canned or frozen vegetables or low-sodium beans, which save time but also preserve nutritional quality. Clean eating is realistic, practical, and conducive to good health and well-being.

The Many Benefits of Going Clean

There are numerous benefits to eating clean. Perhaps most important, when you begin to consume real food and appreciate it for all its textures and flavors, your relationship with it will likely improve and motivate you to continue your journey. Clean eating does not involve giving anything up, but rather savoring the foods that are best for your mind and body.

Weight loss: Because a clean diet includes whole foods with their nutrition intact, it will keep you feeling satisfied on fewer calories. You will likely feel less inclined to snack because your body will be getting all the nutrients it needs to break down the food you eat and sustain your energy throughout the day. Being satiated will lead to fewer snacks, and the positive outcome will be losing weight.

More energy: Research suggests that energy dips and peaks can result from eating processed carbohydrates (such as refined sugars), which are quickly absorbed into the bloodstream, leaving us feeling depleted soon afterward. The unprocessed carbohydrates (often referred to as complex carbs) in whole foods contain fiber and are absorbed more slowly, keeping our energy higher for longer.

Heart health: Clean eating supports optimal heart health. Whole foods are naturally low in sodium and contain monounsaturated and polyunsaturated fats and fiber. The lower sodium is beneficial to blood pressure, and the fat content of whole foods contributes to lowering LDL cholesterol (the bad cholesterol) and raising HDL (good cholesterol). Good cholesterol "cleans" the bad cholesterol from the arteries. Clean eating also includes heart-healthy fats found in foods such as avocados, olive oil, nuts, and seeds, all of which lower LDL cholesterol.

Additionally, the American Heart Association recommends limiting salt intake to about 1 teaspoon per day. Clean eating, which promotes fruits and vegetables, can help make up for the negative effects of sodium with potassium, which counteracts sodium in the body.

Improved mental health: Food fuels not only the body but the brain, too. The choices we make affect the production of the "happy hormones," dopamine and serotonin. A diet rich in healthy fats, including omega-3s from fish, nuts, and avocados, enhances brain function. Diets high in refined sugars and processed foods promote inflammation and decrease insulin sensitivity. The B vitamins found in plant foods also support the production of energy to nourish the brain.

Disease management: A clean-eating lifestyle helps prevent and manage chronic diseases such as diabetes and heart disease. A diet rich in fruits, vegetables, and lean proteins is conducive to achieving and maintaining a healthy weight and decreases the risk of type 2 diabetes. Processed foods contain additives and preservatives, including saturated fats and high levels of salt and sugar, all of which contribute to inflammation, which underlies chronic disease.

Gut health: Diet plays a direct role in gut (digestive tract) health. Studies have shown that there is a relationship between a diet high in processed foods and refined sugars and the health of the microbiome and the production of serotonin. The gut microbiome (naturally occurring bacteria populating our intestines) plays a role in how we digest food, absorb nutrients, and produce nutrients that feed the gut itself. The gut also seems to play roles in food metabolism and immune function. Eating a diverse and well-balanced diet containing unprocessed, wholesome foods can preserve gut health, boost nutrient absorption, and fortify the immune system.

Good, Clean Comfort Food

Comfort foods can certainly be part of clean eating. Once in a while you might want something just the way you've always eaten it. On most occasions you'll swap healthier (and tastier) herbs, spices, and healthy fats for the salt, sugar, and fat. Here are some recipes in this book that might satisfy some of those cravings:

TRADITIONAL COMFORT FOOD	CLEAN EATING ALTERNATIVE
Cheeseburger and French fries	Black-and-White Burgers (page 54); Ultimate Falafel Burgers (page 57); Apple-Sage Turkey Burgers (page 96); Green Bean Fries (page 104)
Beef Chili	Turkey and Butter Bean Chili (page 85); Shepherd's Pie (page 87)
Tacos	Smoky Baja Fish Tacos (page 75); Speedy Steak Fajitas (page 82); Weekend Breakfast Burritos (page 27)
Pizza	Sausage and Broccolini Flatbreads (page 93); No-Crust Pizza Roll-Ups (page 103)
Chocolate Cake	Fudgy Brownies with Date Caramel (page 109); Flourless Oatmeal-Raisin Cookies (page 107); Creamy Banana Mini "Cheesecakes" (page 110)

Fundamentals of Clean Eating

Clean eating is meant to showcase the delicious foods you *can* eat, not those that you can't. In fact, there are no forbidden foods in a clean diet. Remember that the foundation of clean eating is focusing on unprocessed or minimally processed foods (as close to fresh as possible) and reducing the intake of processed foods (those with added ingredients). Here are some of my basic foundations to clean eating to get you started.

Enjoy Nutrient-Dense, Whole Foods

Nutrient-dense foods are as close to their natural state as possible and contain the maximum amounts of vitamins and minerals to support good health. A good rule of thumb for choosing nutrient-dense foods is this: The deeper the color, the more nutritious. Two examples of nutrient-dense foods are kale and salmon. Kale is a deep green cabbage that provides vitamins A and C as well as calcium. Salmon is rich in omega-3 healthy fats. All vegetables, fruits, and lean proteins are considered nutrient dense.

Legumes such as lentils and beans (including canned varieties) are especially nutrient dense. They contain fiber, vitamins, and minerals, including iron, and supply long-lasting energy in the form of complex carbohydrates. Yogurt, particularly plain Greek yogurt, is high in protein and also nutrient dense. And unlike white bread, 100 percent whole-wheat bread has not been stripped of its fiber, vitamins, and minerals. Whole, unprocessed foods sometimes require more preparation and cooking time but are much more nutritious than processed versions.

Foods that are still considered clean, although slightly altered from their most natural forms, include frozen and canned fruits, vegetables, beans, lean meats, and seafood (including canned tuna). These foods can save you time and effort while still providing benefits from their nutrients. Whenever possible, choose fruits without added syrup and look for low-sodium canned foods. Low- and reduced-fat dairy products are also nutrient dense. Refer to the chart Foods to Enjoy, Limit, and Avoid (page 8) to learn more about specific foods that are the best choices.

Leave Processed Foods Behind

Additives such as refined sugar, high-fructose corn syrup, trans fats, and processed vegetable oils have been associated with obesity, type 2 diabetes, and other serious conditions. Hot dogs, cookies, chips, and lunch meats have become everyday foods in the United States. However, many of the synthetic ingredients they contain contribute to chronic conditions, and many have not been thoroughly tested for safety. By leaving processed foods behind as much as possible and focusing on nutrient-dense whole foods, you are putting your health first.

Limit Sugar, Salt, and Oil

Sugar: It's no secret that sugar, especially refined white sugar, contributes to obesity and diabetes. Refined sugar has been linked to inflammation—a main underlying factor for chronic disease. Honey and maple syrup, derived from natural sources, are perhaps the best sweeteners for clean eating. Look for 100 percent pure honey or maple syrup, as these are minimally refined versions. Remember, however, that any natural sweetener still contains calories. A teaspoon or so of a sweetener should be sufficient to sweeten most foods and beverages.

Salt is used as a flavor enhancer and as a preservative. The American Heart Association recommends limiting salt to 2,300 mg per day, which is equal to 1 teaspoon. The Mayo Clinic reports the average American's intake of sodium is closer to 3,400 mg per day! Salt is needed for some essential bodily functions such as for nerves, muscle contractions, and fluid regulation.

I like sea salt and Himalayan salt for their mineral content; however, I use table salt while cooking, which contains iodine, an essential mineral needed for thyroid function.

There are many types of fats and oils, and much confusion over which are healthy and which are harmful. As a rule, solid fats are less healthy than liquid oils. Think about butter and olive oil. Butter is solid and clogs arteries, whereas olive oil flows readily through blood vessels. Avocado is an exception because it is actually a healthy fat. These dietary fats are essential fats, meaning our bodies cannot make them, and we must get them from the foods we consume. Hydrogenated, or "trans," oils and fats have had hydrogen added to them to make them solid (and therefore more shelf stable) and should be avoided.

Choose Quality Whenever Possible

High-quality food is defined as fresh, whole, and nutrient dense. Organic is not always necessary. However, it is recommended for thin-skinned fruits and veggies, like strawberries, raspberries, and tomatoes, that may have been treated with pesticides. When choosing meats and fish, it is important that they are fed a diet that is considered natural for them. If your budget allows it, look for grass-fed, grass-finished beef. Seafood should be wild caught, having eaten a natural diet. I realize organic is expensive; this is where you get to know your local grocery or seafood market and look for sales.

In It for the Long Run

Clean eating is healthy, pleasurable, and incredibly nutritious. It is not a fad diet or a restrictive one but rather it opens up a world of new foods and flavors to explore. It helps us achieve better health, which can enrich and lengthen our lives. Planning, shopping for, preparing, and eating meals with another person can also strengthen communication and fortify the relationship. Sometimes you may find it helpful to write down what you're eating in the beginning of your journey; it helps hold you accountable. Remember, losing weight or changing your lifestyle takes time, but in the long run your weight will stay off and your health conditions will improve. Use this book as a guide and resource to facilitate your adoption of a rewarding new lifestyle.

FOODS TO ENJOY, LIMIT, AND AVOID

	ENJOY	LIMIT	AVOID
FRUIT AND VEGETABLES	All!	None unless you have dietary restrictions	Canned fruits with added sugars or syrups Frozen vegetables in butter and sauces
GRAINS AND LEGUMES	Whole grains (brown rice, quinoa, millet, farro, oatmeal) Chickpeas, lentils, kidney beans, black beans, pinto beans, and navy beans	Whole-wheat pasta Canned beans	Ramen noodles found in packages Boxed mac and cheese, and noodles with Alfredo sauce Beans mixed with dried meats and those with high sodium levels
ANIMAL PROTEIN AND DAIRY	Lean protein (skinless chicken breasts and thighs, grass-fed beef, 90 percent lean ground beef, fish and shellfish, and eggs)	Deli meats (look for ones without nitrates) Canned fish (tuna and salmon)	Canned and processed meats (Spam, chili in a can, hot dogs, and sausages)
DAIRY	Low-fat dairy and nondairy milks, Greek yogurt, kefir (fermented cow's milk), cottage cheese, part-skim mozzarella, and ricotta cheese	Butter, dairy ice cream	Lard, margarine, yogurts with additives and high sugar

NUTS AND SEEDS	Almonds, Brazil nuts, cashews Chia seeds, flaxseed, hemp seeds, pumpkin seeds, sesame seeds, walnuts	Salted nuts and seeds, nut butters	Nuts and seeds covered in sugar and chocolate
FATS AND OILS	Avocado oil, coconut oil, grapeseed oil, olive oil		Refined vegetable oils (corn oil, canola oil), margarine, lard
SWEETENERS, CONDIMENTS, AND SEASONINGS	Whole-grain mustard, dried single spices, vinegars	Honey, maple syrup, molasses Dark chocolate	Refined sugars (white, brown, cane), processed condiments and sauces (e.g., ketchup), dressing/seasoning mix packets (e.g., ranch dressing mix)
BEVERAGES	Water, plain seltzer Herbal teas, filtered coffee without sweeteners, unsweetened nondairy milks, unsweetened lemonade or iced tea	Red wine 100 percent fruit juice Kombucha	Soda and sugary juices like apple juice and some orange juices Alcohol

SHOPPING SAVVY FOR TWO

Shopping for two in supermarkets can be tough. Most supermarkets set up and promote their merchandise for a family of four. Here are some shopping tips to get you through the supermarket without wasting food or breaking your budget.

Plan meals. Planning meals ahead will allow you to reuse fresh ingredients during the week. You can use greens for a salad on Monday and make salads or veggie dishes with those ingredients throughout the week, including for lunch with some added protein or as sides for dinner. Planning will force you to do an inventory of what is in your cabinets, and from there you make a list. This list helps you stay focused in the store and prevents you straying from your list. You end up saving money and not buying random items.

Don't go shopping when you are hungry. If your stomach is growling you tend to shop impulsively and pick up everything that appeals to you, including junk food. Have a snack before shopping to keep temptation away.

Shop at the meat counter. If you eat meat, this can help you choose the exact amount and quality of meat that you need. Butchers often have great tips for preparation as well.

Choose products with the longest shelf life. Check dates on both fresh foods and canned items. For meat, make sure you have a few days to cook it. If not, freeze it immediately for future use.

Shop from the bulk bins. You might think that bulk bins are just for buying large portions of food, but they are great for getting a specific quantity of food. If you need only 1/4 cup of pine nuts for a recipe, check the bulk bins and you just might find exactly the quantity you need.

Let the freezer be your second pantry. Store items that you find on sale and use them later. Purchase meat or chicken in larger packs that can be portioned out and frozen for up to three months. Everything from fresh blueberries, strawberries, corn, and broccoli to milk and bread can be frozen and taken out to enjoy later.

STORAGE TIPS FOR LEFTOVER INGREDIENTS

Being creative with leftovers can decrease your food waste. I know from experience that having leftovers can make me come up with new ideas for the ingredients. In my house, every once in a while, we have a night of "cleaning out the refrigerator" so we don't waste the leftovers or the ingredients we still have on hand, and it can be fun at times. Check out my tips here for common leftover ingredients.

Fresh herbs: Place leftover herbs in a sunny window or on the countertop to thoroughly dry and then store them in a sealed jar or plastic bag, or in the freezer for up to three months.

Stray veggie cuts: Freeze your scraps of veggies like the ends of carrots and celery, mushroom stems, or onion peels for later use. Tie them together in a piece of cheesecloth and place them in soups, or use them to make a homemade stock. They add nutrients and deep flavor.

Lettuce: Wrap leftover lettuce in a damp paper towel or clean kitchen towel and place in the refrigerator to prolong freshness.

Tomato paste: Spread extra paste onto plastic wrap, roll up like a sausage, and freeze.

Beans: Whether you are using canned or dried beans, freeze the cooked leftovers for another dish. Frozen beans can be stored in the freezer for up to six months. They are great on salads or as side dishes.

Crudités: Want some carrots or celery to munch on during the week? Place already-cut veggie sticks in a jar of water, cover, and refrigerate. They'll stay fresh, crisp, and delicious for up to five days.

Pesto: Store leftover pesto (try the recipe on page 114) in ice cube trays. Pop out what you need, thaw, and enjoy for up to six months afterward.

Meal Planning as a Duo

As a former restaurant owner, I know that meal planning is the key to successful clean eating. It has other benefits, too. It helps you:

- Control the portions you prepare and eat
- Budget your time for planning and prepping meals
- Stay within your food budget
- Minimize food waste

Make a list of weekly meals together. Check what foods are in season or on sale to get the freshest food for the best price. Always shop with a list to prevent buying items you don't need.

Plan meals to reuse ingredients and leftovers. In a restaurant, grilled chicken on Monday becomes chicken noodle soup on Wednesday. In planning your weekly meals, try to choose recipes that allow you to use up or reuse key ingredients.

Find common ground. The key to successful and enjoyable clean eating is planning meals that you both love. If you both like chicken, build your week's meals around that key ingredient.

Think outside the box. Variety is the spice of life. Don't get stuck in a rut. Try new recipes and stay open to each other's preferences. A great way to try new tastes is by varying your spices. If you always use salt and pepper on your chicken, try garam masala or za'atar, which can completely transform the taste.

Create a sense of togetherness. Everything from planning your weekly menu to shopping, prepping, and cooking food together can help you feel closer to your partner. Leave room in your menu for ideas and suggestions from both of you. For centuries, stories were passed down through generations when people sat together shucking corn or peeling potatoes. Other stories and family recipes were shared while cooking. Let everything about your meal—from start to finish—create sharing and unity in your home.

LIVE CLEAN, TOO!

Diet is only one piece of living a healthy lifestyle. Clearly, nutrition plays a substantial role in our overall health; however, poor sleep or lack of sleep can have harmful effects, too. Poor sleep can leave us craving sugary snacks, likely because the body is seeking the energy not restored during the night. A helpful tip is to shut off the phone and computer at least a half hour before bedtime. This allows the brain to enter a restful state. Exercise is also a key for health, as it raises the heart rate and produces "happiness hormones," called endorphins. Studies suggest that even minimal bouts of moderate movement can help lower blood sugar and improve heart health. Walking, especially outside, has many health benefits. Sunlight helps maintain vitamin D levels. Walking is also a weight-bearing exercise, which helps maintain healthy bone mass. Even 10 minutes of meditation or yoga can reset your mind and help you relax. The bottom line is that what we eat, how we sleep, and how we move are deeply connected. Making time for all three is key to living a balanced life.

Stocking Your Clean Kitchen

To facilitate your journey to clean eating, here is a list of some of the plant-based staples and helpful equipment you might want for your kitchen and pantry. Many of these items will also be used in the recipes in this book.

Pantry and Counter

Flour: Choose unbleached, all-purpose flour. If you prefer gluten-free, find a gluten-free all-purpose flour such as Bob's Red Mill 1 to 1 Baking Flour.

Grains: Some good grains to have on hand are rice, quinoa, barley, teff, and any others you enjoy.

Legumes: Dried legumes such as lentils, black beans, red kidney beans, and chickpeas are less expensive, but canned versions are nutritionally equivalent. Whenever possible, choose the reduced-sodium varieties.

Nuts and seeds: Purchase raw nuts and seeds and toast them yourself. For maximum shelf life, store in the refrigerator to prevent spoilage.

Oil: When buying oils, look for cold-pressed ones such as avocado and olive oils.

Vinegar: Types such as apple cider, rice, balsamic, and red vinegars are great staples to have on hand for dressings and for adding flavor to dishes.

Honey and/or maple syrup: If your budget allows, look for raw, local honey and 100 percent pure maple syrup. Darker maple syrup contains more minerals and antioxidants.

Dried fruit: Dried fruit such as raisins, cranberries, and dates can naturally sweeten dishes. Look for unsweetened and unsulfured fruit for the healthiest options.

Soy sauce/tamari: Look for lower-sodium soy sauce or tamari. Tamari is a gluten-free soy sauce, so it is perfect for anyone avoiding gluten.

Alliums: Alliums such as onions and garlic are great to have on hand to add an enormous amount of flavor to dishes. Look for onions and garlic that have not begun to sprout (growing offshoots) and are free from any soft spots.

Root vegetables: When purchasing root vegetables such as sweet potatoes, beets, potatoes, carrots, turnips, onions, and radishes, look for ones that are firm and free of any soft spots and sprouting. Beets are best with the greens still attached; then you know they are fresh, and as an added bonus, you can sauté the greens as an additional vegetable.

Dried spices: Check the date on spices when purchasing to ensure that they will not expire within a year. Buy small amounts so they don't expire before you use them.

Salt and pepper: Today, regular white salt is one of many salts on the market. Sea salt and Himalayan salt offer different minerals. Experiment with them to add nutrition and new tastes to dishes.

Refrigerator and Freezer

Eggs: When buying eggs, look for pasture-raised, cage-free organic eggs if your budget allows. Always be sure to check the package for any cracks or leakage.

Milk/nondairy milk: When buying dairy milk, look for grass-fed, organic milk. For nondairy milk, look for a brand that contains a small number of ingredients. Always check the expiration date.

Leafy green vegetables: Leafy greens such as spinach, kale, and collard greens add a wealth of vitamins and minerals to your plate. Look for bright green leaves free from yellow spots or visible discoloration. If your budget allows, purchase organic.

Nonstarchy vegetables: When purchasing nonstarchy vegetables such as bell peppers, cabbage, broccoli, Brussels sprouts, summer squash, and green beans, test the produce for firmness, bruises, and soft spots. If your budget allows, buy organic.

Fresh fruit: Because it's usually fresher and cheaper, buy fruit that's in season. For example, berries and melons are much cheaper in the summer than in the winter. Bananas are an excellent fruit to buy year-round.

Frozen fruits and vegetables: Look for frozen fruits and vegetables that contain no added ingredients such as sauces or syrups. Frozen fruits and vegetables can actually be high in nutrients because they are picked at peak ripeness and flash frozen.

Avocados: Find those that are slightly soft and dark in color with no obvious signs of damage. A great way to make sure a soft avocado is at peak ripeness is to remove the small bit of stem at the top of the fruit. A ripe fruit will have green, not brown, flesh. If you plan to use the avocados in three to four days, pick ones that are firm, still have their bit of stem, and are brighter green. To accelerate ripening, place avocados in a paper bag.

Herbs: Opt for organic herbs such as cilantro, parsley, and rosemary. Trim the ends of tender herbs like cilantro and parsley and keep in a jar of water in the refrigerator, changing the water every couple of days. Wrap woody herbs like thyme or rosemary in a damp paper towel and put them in a container to chill in the refrigerator.

Citrus: Citrus is a crucial ingredient for bringing acidity and flavor to dishes. Lemons, limes, and oranges are great to have on hand. If using the peel (such as to make a zest), buy organic if possible.

Frozen fish/shellfish: Look for wild-caught fish and shellfish if possible. Buying frozen fish will help cut costs, especially when it is on sale. Avoid any fish with signs of ice crystals or discoloration.

Kitchen Equipment List

- 2-quart and 4-quart saucepans
- 8- or 10-inch nonstick skillet or sauté pan
- Rimmed baking sheet
- Muffin tin
- Mixing bowls (stainless steel or glass)
- Measuring cups and measuring spoons
- Food processor (with grater and slicer attachments, if possible)
- Cutting board
- Chef's knife and paring knife
- Mixing spoons, spatula, whisk
- Colander
- Parchment paper

About the Recipes

I believe you will enjoy my recipes in this book, all of which are based on a clean-eating plan for two. They call for fresh and minimally processed ingredients. The nutrition information at the end of each recipe will help reassure you that you are getting balanced nutrition without the synthetic ingredients that detract from good taste.

Easy Recipes for Two

Keep in mind that I have chosen three quick cooking methods for all of the recipes:

One Pot: Every recipe with this label is made with ingredients that go into the same cooking vessel. This can be a pot, skillet, or even a baking sheet. Using only one vessel saves time not only in cooking but also in cleaning up.

5-Ingredient: A recipe made with five ingredients or fewer is a boon when you are time strapped. You'll save time shopping, prepping, and cooking. It's important to note that this does not count any water, cooking oil/spray, or salt and pepper in the five ingredients.

Quick: These meals can be prepped and cooked in 30 minutes or less. You can trim off even more prep time by washing and chopping your vegetables as soon as you get home from the market. The French call this "mise en place," which means having everything in place.

Recipe Help

The recipes are labeled appropriately for certain dietary needs, including gluten-free, dairy-free, vegan, and vegetarian. This will make it easy to find the recipes that are right for you. The recipes also include tips to help you get the most out of each one:

Cooking tip: These tips will give guidance on how to make meal prep and cooking easier and more streamlined.

Substitution tip: These offer alternative ingredients so you can tailor the recipe to your own taste preferences or dietary needs.

Variation tip: I'll provide variation options for times you may not have a certain ingredient on hand or want to swap something out.

Use it up: These are ideas for how to use up purchased ingredients or leftovers. In some cases, I'll even point to other recipes in this book!

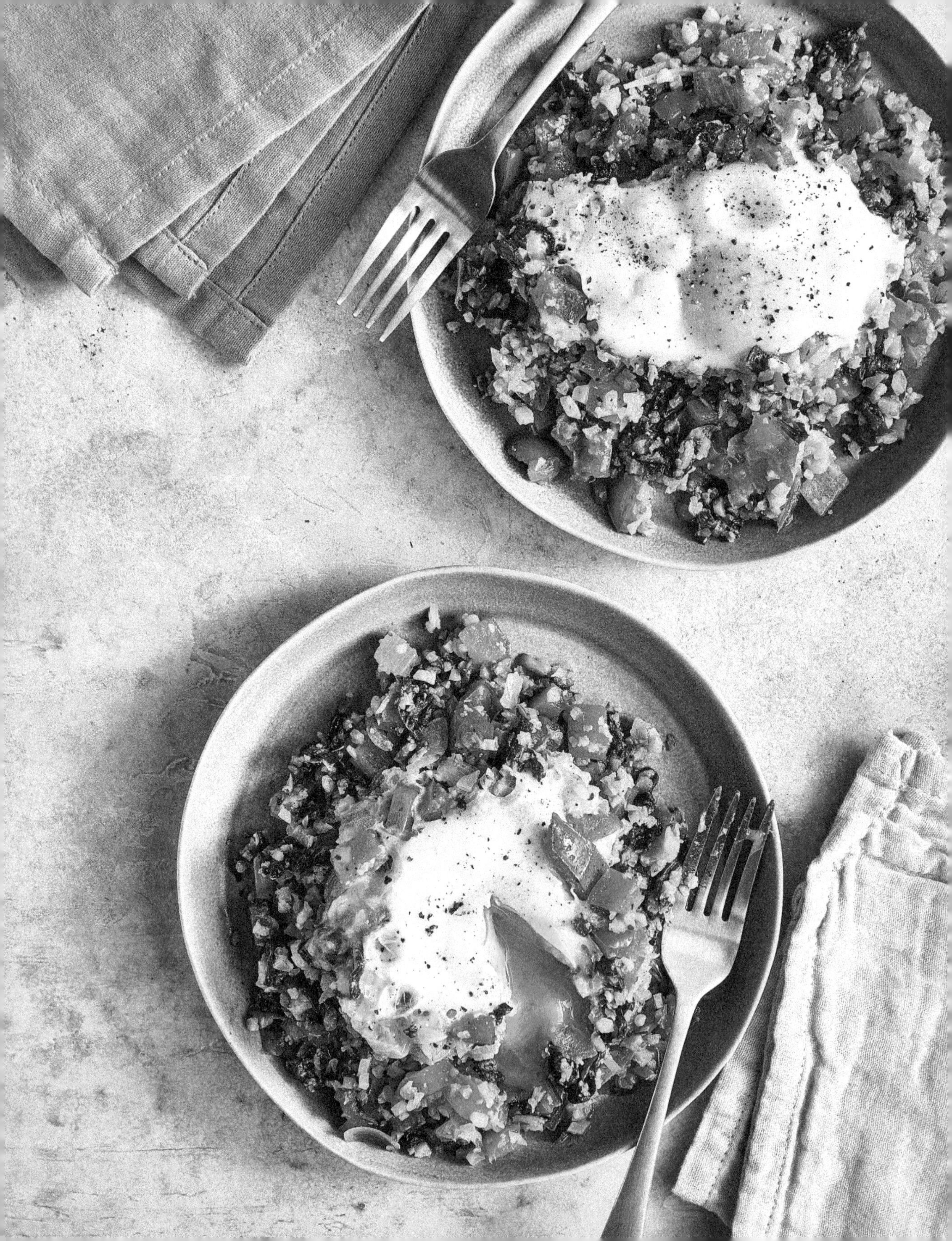

CHAPTER TWO

Breakfast and Brunch

Bird's Nest Cauliflower Eggs

Prep time: 10 minutes | Cook time: 10 minutes | Serves: 2

Quick, One Pot, Gluten-Free, Vegetarian

What beats eggs and vegetables to start your day? Cauliflower contains sulfur, which helps with removing toxins from the body, making it perfect breakfast fare. Also with spinach and tomatoes, this is one nutrient-packed meal that you will want to make again and again.

- 3 teaspoons olive oil, divided
- ¼ cup chopped sweet onion
- ¼ cup chopped red bell pepper
- 1 small garlic clove, minced
- ½ teaspoon dried oregano
- ½ teaspoon salt, plus more for seasoning
- ¼ teaspoon paprika
- 1½ cups cauliflower rice
- 1½ teaspoons freshly squeezed lemon juice
- 5 ounces frozen spinach, thawed and well drained, or fresh spinach, chopped
- ½ cup chopped plum tomato
- ½ cup shredded Cheddar cheese
- 2 large eggs
- Freshly ground black pepper

1. In an 8-inch nonstick skillet or sauté pan, heat 2 teaspoons of oil over medium heat and swirl to coat the pan.
2. Add the onion, bell pepper, and garlic, and cook for about 2 minutes, until the onion begins to soften. Add the oregano, salt, and paprika, and stir.
3. Add the cauliflower rice and the remaining 1 teaspoon of oil, and cook, stirring frequently, for 1 to 2 minutes. Add the lemon juice and stir, then add the spinach and tomato and stir to incorporate all the ingredients.
4. Sprinkle the cheese evenly over the mixture and gently make two wells, one for each egg. Crack the eggs into the wells, cover, and cook for about 7 minutes for runny eggs, or longer for firmer yolks.
5. Season with additional salt and pepper. Divide the cauliflower mixture and place 1 egg on each plate to serve.

SUBSTITUTION TIP: Feel free to change out the Cheddar for your favorite cheese or omit altogether to make this dairy-free.

Per serving: Calories: 313; Fat: 21g; Sodium: 912mg; Carbohydrates: 13g; Fiber: 5g; Sugar: 5g; Protein: 18g

Bibimbap

Prep time: 5 minutes | Cook time: 5 minutes | Serves: 2

Quick, One Pot, Gluten-Free, Vegetarian

Bibimbap is a traditional Korean rice dish often topped with kimchi. In this version, sauerkraut is used because it's tasty and provides the same probiotic health benefits as kimchi. This breakfast is a great way to use up any extra rice or greens in your refrigerator.

- 4 teaspoons butter, divided
- 2 scallions, both white and green parts, chopped
- 1½ cups cooked brown rice
- 5 or 6 kale leaves or any leafy green of choice, chopped
- 1 tablespoon water, if needed
- ½ cup sauerkraut
- 2 large eggs
- Sesame oil, for serving
- Tamari, for serving

1. In a skillet or sauté pan, melt 2 teaspoons of butter over medium heat. Add the scallions and cook until bright green. Add the cooked rice and heat through. Push the rice off to one side of the pan.
2. Add the remaining 2 teaspoons of butter to the pan and add the greens, cooking until tender and soft, about 30 seconds. If needed, add 1 tablespoon of water.
3. In the third section of the pan, add the sauerkraut and heat through.
4. Divide the rice between two bowls and top each with half of the greens and sauerkraut. In the same skillet, crack the eggs into the pan. Once the whites of the eggs begin to set, flip them over. Cook until the yolks reach the desired doneness.
5. Place the eggs over the rice, greens, and sauerkraut, and dress the bowls with drizzles of sesame oil and tamari.

COOKING TIP: You can add more toppings onto the bowl such as shredded carrots, sesame seeds, apple cider vinegar, or sriracha.

Per serving: Calories: 361; Fat: 14g; Sodium: 375mg; Carbohydrates: 46g; Fiber: 4.5g; Sugar: 1.5g; Protein: 12g

Blueberry Breakfast Muffins

Prep time: 10 minutes | Cook time: 20 minutes | Makes: 4 muffins

This is one of my family's favorite muffin recipes. Blueberries contain antioxidants, which help reduce inflammation and are heart healthy. These muffins have protein from the yogurt, and less sugar than store-bought ones. They are great to have year-round, and you can use frozen berries instead of the fresh ones. Make a double batch and keep the extras in the freezer for another day.

- ½ cup all-purpose flour
- ¾ teaspoon baking powder
- Pinch salt
- 1 large egg
- ¼ cup honey
- 1 tablespoon butter, melted
- ¼ cup plus 1 tablespoon plain low-fat Greek yogurt
- ⅓ cup blueberries
- ¼ teaspoon grated lemon zest

1. Preheat the oven to 375°F. Line four wells of a muffin tin with muffin liners or parchment paper.
2. In a medium bowl, combine the flour, baking powder, and salt.
3. In a separate bowl, beat the egg and then add the honey and whisk vigorously. Add the melted butter slowly while whisking. Add half the yogurt at a time, mixing until just combined. Mix in the blueberries and lemon zest.
4. Using a spatula, fold the wet ingredients into the dry ingredients until the batter comes together. Divide the batter between the four wells of the muffin tin and bake for 20 minutes or until the muffins are golden brown and a toothpick comes out clean from the center.

SUBSTITUTION TIP: For a slightly different fruit flavor, substitute fresh or frozen raspberries or strawberries for the blueberries.

Per serving (2 muffins): Calories: 370; Fat: 9.5g; Sodium: 206mg; Carbohydrates: 64g; Fiber: 1.5g; Sugar: 36g; Protein: 10g

Simple Smashed Breakfast Hash

Prep time: 10 minutes | Cook time: 10 minutes | Serves: 2

Quick, Dairy-Free, Gluten-Free, Vegetarian

Sweet potato is packed with fiber and antioxidants, which are great for gut health and for fighting chronic diseases. This vegetarian breakfast will surprise you by how filling it is, and it's oh so quick to prepare. You will be eating before your coffee is even finished brewing.

---

1 medium sweet potato
1 small zucchini
1 small yellow squash
1 tablespoon olive oil
3 ounces shiitake, white button, or cremini mushrooms, sliced
1 shallot, chopped
¼ teaspoon salt, plus more if needed
¼ teaspoon freshly ground black pepper, plus more if needed
2 to 4 large eggs

1. Cook the sweet potato in the microwave for 4 to 5 minutes until soft, being careful not to overcook. While the sweet potato is cooking, cut the zucchini and squash lengthwise and then lengthwise again, ending up with four long pieces. Cut the long pieces into ½-inch pieces.
2. In a nonstick skillet or sauté pan, heat the oil over medium heat and swirl to coat. Add the zucchini, squash, mushrooms, and shallot, and cook until the zucchini and squash begin to soften and the edges turn golden, about 5 minutes. Season with the salt and pepper.
3. When the veggies are almost cooked, heat a separate nonstick pan over medium heat, crack the eggs into the pan, and cook for 3 minutes for soft yolks, or longer for firmer yolks.
4. Cut the cooked sweet potato in half and place one half on the center of each plate. Cut the sweet potato crosswise and smash with a potato masher or a fork. Place the cooked veggies over the sweet potato and top with the eggs. Season with more salt and pepper if needed.

VARIATION TIP: You can substitute a white or red potato for the sweet potato.

USE IT UP: Wrap up the leftover shallot and mushrooms to use later for another dish. This is a great way to use up leftover squash or mushrooms in your refrigerator.

Per serving (with 2 eggs): Calories: 308; Fat: 17g; Sodium: 481mg; Carbohydrates: 24g; Fiber: 5g; Sugar: 8.5g; Protein: 16g

Mini Crustless Spinach and Sweet Potato Tarts

Prep time: 10 minutes | Cook time: 20 minutes | Makes: 4 mini tarts

Quick, Gluten-Free, Vegetarian

These mini tarts are perfect for those mornings when you are in a hurry. Using an ice cream scoop is a great way to measure the mixture out into the muffin tins evenly, and using a muffin liner makes cleanup easier. These are great for on-the-go, but if you have time to enjoy them at home, serve on a bed of lettuce with a bowl of fruit.

- Olive oil, for greasing
- 1 medium (5-ounce) sweet potato
- 2 large eggs plus 1 large egg white
- ¼ teaspoon salt
- ¼ teaspoon freshly ground black pepper
- ⅓ cup chopped spinach
- ¼ cup half and half
- 1 teaspoon chopped scallion
- 1 tablespoon grated Parmesan cheese (check label for vegetarian)
- 1 tablespoon crumbled goat cheese
- Lettuce, for serving (optional)
- Cantaloupe slices, for serving (optional)

1. Preheat the oven to 350°F. Grease four wells of a muffin tin with oil.
2. Cook the sweet potato in the microwave for 4 to 5 minutes, until soft. While the potato is cooking, in a medium bowl, whisk the eggs and egg white, and season with the salt and pepper. Add the spinach, half and half, and scallion, and mix to combine. Mash the sweet potato and add to the mixture. Stir in the Parmesan cheese and goat cheese.
3. Divide the mixture evenly between the four prepared wells of the muffin tin and bake for 20 minutes or until the center is cooked through. Serve over a bed of lettuce with a side of cantaloupe slices, if using.

VARIATION TIP: If you don't have spinach, use another green like arugula or kale. Substitute shallot or sweet onion for the scallion. The cheese can be easily replaced with whatever you have in your refrigerator. Feel free to add turmeric or other herbs.

Per serving (2 mini tarts): Calories: 280; Fat: 19g; Sodium: 511mg; Carbohydrates: 16g; Fiber: 2g; Sugar: 4.5g; Protein: 12g

Golden Spiced Granola

Prep time: 5 minutes | Cook time: 25 minutes | Serves: 2

Turmeric is not only anti-inflammatory, but it also gives this granola its golden color. It may seem odd to mix in some black pepper, but black pepper contains a compound called "piperine," which helps enhance the absorption of curcumin, the active compound in turmeric.

- ¼ cup rolled oats
- 2 tablespoons raw almonds, chopped
- 1 tablespoon raw pumpkin seeds
- 1 tablespoon unsweetened or juice-sweetened dried cranberries
- 1 tablespoon unsweetened shredded coconut
- ¼ teaspoon ground cinnamon
- ⅛ teaspoon ground cardamom
- ⅛ teaspoon ground ginger
- ⅛ teaspoon ground turmeric
- Pinch salt
- Pinch freshly ground black pepper
- 2 tablespoons maple syrup
- 1 tablespoon coconut oil, melted

1. Preheat the oven to 325°F.
2. In a bowl, combine the oats, almonds, pumpkin seeds, cranberries, coconut, cinnamon, cardamom, ginger, turmeric, salt, and pepper, and mix well to evenly distribute.
3. Add the maple syrup and coconut oil and stir to combine until everything is coated. Line a baking sheet with parchment paper and spread the mixture evenly in one layer.
4. Bake for 20 to 25 minutes or until golden brown, mixing halfway through. Allow the granola to cool on the baking sheet before enjoying.

VARIATION TIP: You can use whatever nuts or seeds you have on hand, such as pecans, cashews, or sunflower seeds.

SUBSTITUTION TIP: To make this recipe gluten-free, be sure to purchase certified gluten-free oats.

Per serving Calories: 241; Fat: 14g; Sodium: 148mg; Carbohydrates: 26g; Fiber: 2.5g; Sugar: 15g; Protein: 4g

Sunday Morning Pancakes

Prep time: 10 minutes | Cook time: 5 minutes | Serves: 2

I love these pancakes for the added protein and heart-healthy flaxseed, and they will keep you feeling full longer than boxed pancakes. Add a sunny-side up egg or scrambled eggs to bring the diner experience right to your kitchen. Top with maple syrup and fresh fruit (blueberries are my favorite) to complete the dish. Make them gluten-free by trading out the flour for your favorite gluten-free variety. They can also be made dairy-free by using a coconut-based yogurt.

- ¾ cup whole-wheat or gluten-free flour
- 1½ tablespoons ground flaxseed
- 1 teaspoon baking powder
- ¼ teaspoon baking soda
- Pinch salt
- ½ cup plain low-fat Greek yogurt
- ½ cup water
- 1 small banana (3 to 4 ounces), mashed
- 1 large egg
- 2 tablespoons olive oil, plus more for greasing

1. In a medium bowl, combine the flour, ground flaxseed, baking powder, baking soda, and salt, and mix well.
2. In a separate bowl, combine the yogurt, water, banana, egg, and oil, and mix well. Make a well in the dry ingredients and pour in the wet ingredients slowly. Stir until just combined.
3. Lightly oil a skillet or griddle with oil and heat over medium to high heat. Ladle ⅓ cup of batter onto the heated pan for each pancake. Cook until bubbles appear on top, 1 to 2 minutes. Turn the pancakes over and cook on the second side until golden brown, about 1 minute. You may need to cook them in batches.

VARIATION TIP: If you need these to be gluten-free, you can change out the flour for Bob's Red Mill All-Purpose Gluten-Free Flour or a similar blend, and they will still taste great.

USE IT UP: Need just one serving? Cook the rest of the batter, let cool, and freeze the pancakes in a container.

Per serving: Calories: 461; Fat: 23g; Sodium: 619mg; Carbohydrates: 51g; Fiber: 7.5g; Sugar: 8.5g; Protein: 16g

Weekend Breakfast Burritos

Prep time: 10 minutes | Cook time: 10 minutes | Serves: 2

Quick, Gluten-Free, Vegetarian

Who doesn't like a burrito, right? This is also a great alternative to a bacon and egg sandwich. Corn tortilla wraps are available at most supermarkets. I love easy recipes with robust flavors that come together. Serve these with fresh fruit for breakfast, or any time of day.

- ½ teaspoon olive oil
- ¼ cup diced green bell pepper
- ¼ cup diced sweet onion
- 1 small plum tomato, diced (about ½ cup)
- 4 large eggs
- ¼ cup reduced-fat milk or unsweetened almond milk
- ¼ teaspoon salt
- ⅛ teaspoon freshly ground black pepper
- 2 (10-inch) corn tortilla wraps

1. In a medium skillet, heat the oil over medium heat and cook the bell pepper and onion for 1 to 2 minutes, until soft. Add the tomato and stir to combine.
2. In a medium bowl, whisk the eggs, milk, salt, and pepper. Pour the egg mixture over the vegetables and cook for 4 to 5 minutes to the desired doneness.
3. Divide the mixture between the two tortillas. To wrap the burrito, fold the two ends into the middle and then wrap the bottom over the egg mixture and two ends, and roll.

USE IT UP: Cover leftover tortilla wraps in plastic wrap and freeze for up to 3 months.

Per serving: Calories: 246; Fat: 12g; Sodium: 465mg; Carbohydrates: 19g; Fiber: 3g; Sugar: 5g; Protein: 15g

Easy Avocado Toast

Prep time: 5 minutes | Cook time: 5 minutes | Serves: 2

This is the quintessential avocado toast and can be loaded up with your favorite toppings. Avocado is a healthy fat that will keep you feeling full. You may want to add a third slice of bread to share because the dish is so tasty. This is a perfect grab-and-go toast if you are in a hurry.

2 slices bread of choice
1 avocado, peeled and pitted
¼ lemon
1 teaspoon olive oil, for drizzling
⅛ teaspoon salt
⅛ teaspoon freshly ground black pepper

1. Toast the bread.
2. In a small bowl, mash the avocado and spread half of it on each slice. Top with a squeeze of lemon, a drizzle of oil, and the salt and pepper.
3. You can eat the toast as is, or add any desired toppings, including but not limited to the ones listed in the tip. You can really make this your own and use whatever you have on hand.

SUBSTITUTION TIP: To make this gluten-free, use your favorite gluten-free bread.

VARIATION TIP: Try these other toppings to change it up: fried egg or sliced hard-boiled egg; radishes, red onion, or cucumber, thinly sliced; arugula, spinach, or sprouts; pumpkin, sesame, or sunflower seeds; feta or goat cheese; smoked salmon; red pepper flakes, sumac, or other spice of choice.

Per serving: Calories: 225; Fat: 14g; Sodium: 341mg; Carbohydrates: 23g; Fiber: 6.5g; Sugar: 2.5g; Protein: 6g

Toast Points with Cottage Cheese

Prep time: 5 minutes | Cook time: 5 minutes | Serves: 2

Quick, 5-Ingredient, One Pot, Vegetarian

I never liked cottage cheese until I created this recipe and found out I actually love it. My favorite brand is Good Culture cottage cheese. It's a clean product with 8 grams of protein, which helps me feel full until lunchtime. Get creative with the toppings and enjoy this with your morning coffee or tea. It's also a great on-the-run breakfast.

- 4 slices whole-wheat bread
- 1 cup low-fat cottage cheese
- 1½ plum tomatoes, cut into about 6 slices
- ¼ cucumber, cut into about 6 slices
- 1 teaspoon olive oil, for drizzling
- ¼ teaspoon salt
- ⅛ teaspoon freshly ground black pepper

Toast the bread. Top the bread with the cottage cheese, the tomato and cucumber slices, and a drizzle of oil. Season with the salt and pepper. Cut each slice in half.

VARIATION TIP: You can add additional toppings such as red onion, avocado, and smoked salmon.

Per serving: Calories: 363; Fat: 8g; Sodium: 942mg; Carbohydrates: 50g; Fiber: 4.5g; Sugar: 14g; Protein: 20g

Pecan-Cinnamon Breakfast Quinoa

Prep time: 5 minutes | Cook time: 10 minutes | Serves: 2

When I get tired of oatmeal but want something warm, this quinoa bowl does the trick. Did you know quinoa is a great source of fiber and protein? Using leftover quinoa is not only a great way to use it up, but it makes this a quick breakfast. For toppings, I recommend hemp seeds, dried fruit, nutmeg, cinnamon, or even coconut milk or a bit of yogurt.

- 4 tablespoons pecans, chopped
- 3 teaspoons avocado oil
- 1 teaspoon ground cinnamon
- Pinch salt
- 2 cups cooked quinoa
- 2 tablespoons honey

1. In a small saucepan, toast the pecans over medium heat, stirring often until they become fragrant, 4 to 6 minutes.
2. Add the avocado oil, cinnamon, and salt to the saucepan and stir for about 10 seconds, then add the cooked quinoa. Mix until everything is fully incorporated and the quinoa is heated through.
3. Remove the saucepan from the heat and stir in the honey.
4. Divide the mixture between two bowls and top with your choice of toppings. Serve promptly.

COOKING TIP: Quinoa is a great staple to have on hand. When making recipes with quinoa, such as Spring Vegetable Quinoa Salad (page 42), you can make larger batches and then cool and freeze the quinoa in freezer-safe containers for later use. You can also find precooked quinoa in the freezer section at the grocery store.

SUBSTITUTION TIP: To make this nut-free, you can substitute pumpkin or sunflower seeds for the pecans. To make this vegan, swap maple syrup for the honey.

Per serving: Calories: 442; Fat: 20g; Sodium: 159mg; Carbohydrates: 58g; Fiber: 6.5g; Sugar: 18g; Protein: 9g

Chickpea Breakfast Pita Pocket

Prep time: 5 minutes | Cook time: 5 minutes | Serves: 2

Chickpeas are so versatile that I try to always keep them in my pantry. I love a boiled egg squashed in a pita pocket, so for this recipe, I switched it up and used mashed chickpeas. You could also add cheese if you are not following a vegan diet. There's plenty of room to add other spices, too, like maybe a little hot sauce to spice it up a bit.

1 tablespoon olive oil
2 tablespoons chopped onion
2 tablespoons chopped red bell pepper
¼ teaspoon ground turmeric
¼ teaspoon paprika
¼ teaspoon salt
Freshly ground black pepper
1 cup canned chickpeas, drained, rinsed, and mashed
1 cup chopped spinach or arugula
2 tablespoons water
2 whole-wheat pitas

1. In a nonstick skillet or sauté pan, heat the oil over medium heat and sauté the onion and bell pepper for 1 to 2 minutes, until the onion begins to soften. Add the turmeric and paprika, and season with the salt and pepper. Cook until fragrant. Stir in the mashed chickpeas to combine. Add the spinach and water and cook for 1 to 2 minutes, until the spinach wilts.
2. Cut the pitas in half and fill each half with one-quarter of the mixture.

COOKING TIP: The chickpea mixture freezes well, so feel free to make extra and save some for a quick breakfast on a hectic morning.

VARIATION TIP: To increase the protein, you can add 4 ounces of ground chicken and sauté with the onion and pepper. Change the greens to whatever you have in the house.

Per serving: Calories: 315; Fat: 8.5g; Sodium: 695mg; Carbohydrates: 47g; Fiber: 7.5g; Sugar: 4g; Protein: 13g

Carrot Cake Oatmeal

Prep time: 10 minutes | Cook time: 20 minutes | Serves: 2

Quick, Vegan

This recipe transforms regular oatmeal into a delicious, healthy breakfast. Adding vegetables to your breakfast is a great way to pack in micronutrients early in the day. Carrots are high in vitamin A, fiber, and potassium and have been linked to lower cholesterol levels and improved eye health.

- 1½ cups water
- ½ cup steel-cut oats
- Pinch salt
- 2 tablespoons walnut halves
- 1 cup finely grated carrot
- ¼ cup raisins
- 1 teaspoon ground cinnamon
- ⅛ teaspoon ground ginger
- ⅛ teaspoon ground allspice
- Pinch ground nutmeg
- 2 tablespoons maple syrup

1. In a 4-quart saucepan, bring the water to a boil over high heat. Add the oats and salt and reduce the heat to medium-low and cook for 10 minutes, stirring frequently.
2. While the oats are cooking, in a small skillet, toast the walnuts over medium-low heat for 3 to 4 minutes, until fragrant. Remove from the heat to let cool. Once cooled, coarsely chop the walnuts and set aside.
3. Once almost all the water has been absorbed by the oats, add the carrot, raisins, cinnamon, ginger, allspice, and nutmeg, and stir to combine. Continue to cook until the oats have fully thickened, about 5 more minutes.
4. Take the oats off the heat and stir in the maple syrup. Divide between two bowls and top with the chopped nuts.

VARIATION TIP: You can swap dried cranberries for the raisins, or another nut of choice for the walnuts. You can also change up the spices to create your own version. Use what you have on hand.

SUBSTITUTION TIP: To make this recipe gluten-free, make sure to buy certified gluten-free oats. Omit the nuts to make this nut-free.

Per serving: Calories: 327; Fat: 7g; Sodium: 188mg; Carbohydrates: 63g; Fiber: 6.5g; Sugar: 28g; Protein: 7g

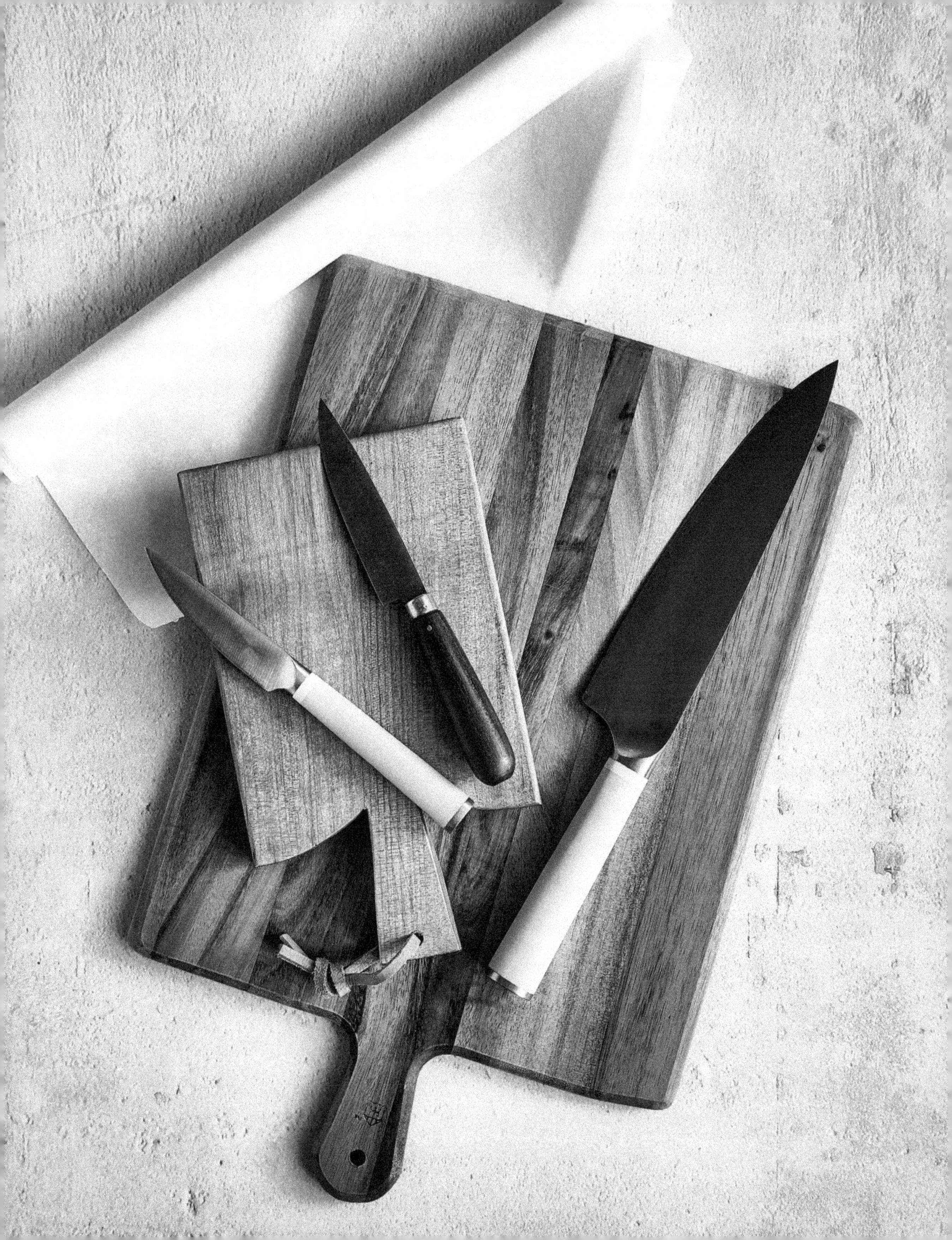

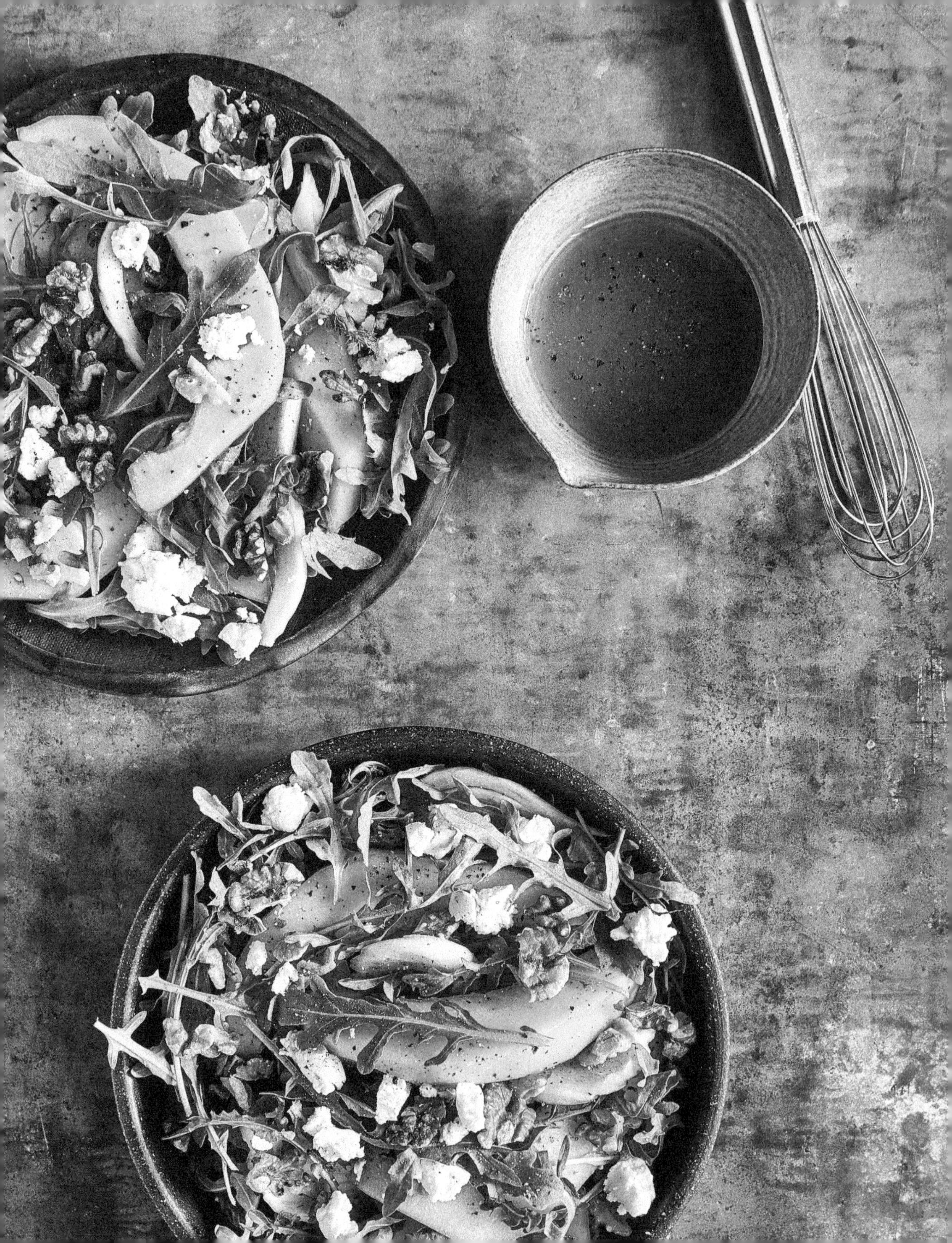

CHAPTER THREE

Soups, Salads, and Sandwiches

Arugula, Fennel, and Cantaloupe Salad

Prep time: 10 minutes | Cook time: 5 minutes | Serves: 2

This refreshing salad can be eaten as a first course before a main dish or as a meal with a side of grilled fish or grilled chicken. The flavors are a nice blend of bitter and sweet. The arugula and cantaloupe are low in calories, but both are high in vitamin C, a powerful antioxidant to fight off inflammation and chronic disease. And let's not forget the fiber content in this salad.

- 1 cantaloupe, peeled and thinly cut into about 16 slices
- 5 cups loosely packed arugula
- 1 cup thinly sliced fennel
- ½ cup walnuts
- ½ cup crumbled goat cheese
- 1 tablespoon olive oil
- 1 teaspoon freshly squeezed lemon juice
- ⅛ teaspoon salt
- ⅛ teaspoon freshly ground black pepper

1. Divide the cantaloupe, arugula, and fennel between two plates.
2. In a small skillet or sauté pan, toast the walnuts for 1 to 2 minutes over low heat, until fragrant. Once cool, coarsely chop the walnuts and divide them between each plate along with the goat cheese.
3. In a small bowl, mix the oil and lemon juice and season with the salt and pepper. Drizzle half of the dressing over each plate.

VARIATION TIP: Use another nut such as almonds, or if you have an allergy, pumpkin seeds work well in place of the nuts.

USE IT UP: If you have extra arugula, you can use it in the Chickpea Breakfast Pita Pocket (page 31).

Per serving: Calories: 469; Fat: 34g; Sodium: 377mg; Carbohydrates: 31g; Fiber: 6g; Sugar: 24g; Protein: 16g

Bell Pepper and Chickpea Salad

Prep time: 10 minutes | Serves: 2

Quick, Dairy-Free, Gluten-Free, Vegetarian

This bright Mediterranean-style salad was inspired by a trip to Greece. It's great alone or served with grilled chicken or salmon. Grilled octopus would also make a great accompaniment for a summer dinner if you can buy fresh seafood. Packed with fiber and plant-based protein, this salad has flavors that will leave you wanting more.

For the salad

1 (15-ounce) can chickpeas, drained and rinsed
½ cup chopped red bell pepper
½ cup chopped green bell pepper
10 cherry tomatoes, halved
2 tablespoons chopped red onion
2 tablespoons chopped fresh cilantro

For the dressing

2 tablespoons olive oil
1½ tablespoons freshly squeezed lemon juice
½ teaspoon honey
½ teaspoon salt
⅛ teaspoon freshly ground black pepper

To make the salad

1. In a bowl, combine the chickpeas, bell peppers, cherry tomatoes, red onion, and cilantro.

To make the dressing

2. In a jar, combine the oil, lemon juice, and honey. Season with the salt and pepper and shake well to mix. Divide the chickpea mixture between two plates and pour the dressing evenly over each salad. Toss to coat.

USE IT UP: Have leftover red bell pepper and fresh cilantro? Use them in the Spring Vegetable Quinoa Salad (page 42).

Per serving: Calories: 323; Fat: 17g; Sodium: 831mg; Carbohydrates: 36g; Fiber: 10g; Sugar: 11g; Protein: 10g

Creamy Vegetable Soup

Prep time: 10 minutes | Cook time: 15 minutes | Serves: 2

This soup is perfect no matter the season. I love the contrast of sweetness from the butternut squash and bitterness from the parsnips. The coconut milk creates a creamy, velvety texture, and nutmeg balances the flavors perfectly. For a bigger meal, serve this soup with the Spring Vegetable Quinoa Salad (page 42), which is also vegan and gluten-free, to make this a complete meal.

1½ teaspoons olive oil
1 onion, diced
1 carrot, diced
⅛ teaspoon ground nutmeg
1 cup diced butternut squash
¾ cup diced parsnip
1¼ cups vegetable broth
½ cup water
¼ cup canned light coconut milk
½ teaspoon salt
¼ teaspoon freshly ground black pepper

1. In a 4-quart pot, heat the oil over medium heat and swirl to coat. Add the onion and carrot and cook for about 5 minutes, until the onion becomes translucent and the carrot begins to soften. Season with the nutmeg.
2. Add the butternut squash and parsnip, mixing to incorporate. Pour in the vegetable broth and water and bring the mixture to a boil. Reduce the heat to low, cover, and let simmer until all the vegetables have softened and are cooked through, about 10 minutes.
3. Turn off the heat and carefully blend using an immersion blender or potato masher. You can also use a regular blender, blending in two batches if needed. Add the coconut milk and season with the salt and pepper.

USE IT UP: You might have leftover butternut squash that you can roast with a little olive oil and use as a side with dinner tonight or tomorrow.

Per serving: Calories: 164; Fat: 5g; Sodium: 636mg; Carbohydrates: 29g; Fiber: 6.5g; Sugar: 9.5g; Protein: 3g

Hearty Kale and Bean Chicken Soup

Prep time: 10 minutes | Cook time: 20 minutes | Serves: 2

Quick, Dairy-Free, Gluten-Free

Loaded with protein from the beans and chicken and fiber from the kale, carrots, and beans, this soup can be a hearty meal on its own. If you're looking for a bit more for your meal, the Kale and Apple Salad (page 40) would make a great choice. Both are quick, simple, and tasty.

- 7 ounces boneless, skinless chicken thighs
- ¾ teaspoon salt, divided
- Freshly ground black pepper
- 1 tablespoon olive oil
- ½ cup chopped onion
- 1 carrot, chopped
- 1 thyme sprig
- 1 garlic clove, crushed
- ⅛ teaspoon red pepper flakes
- 2½ cups low-sodium chicken broth
- 1 (15-ounce) can white kidney beans, drained and rinsed
- 1 cup chopped kale

1. Preheat the oven to 375°F.
2. Place the chicken on a baking sheet and season with ½ teaspoon of salt and the pepper. Bake for about 15 minutes or until a thermometer inserted in the thickest part reaches 165°F.
3. While the chicken is baking, in a 4-quart saucepan, heat the oil over medium heat, swirling to coat the pan. Add the onion, carrot, thyme sprig, garlic, remaining ¼ teaspoon of salt, and the red pepper flakes and cook for 3 minutes, stirring occasionally, until the onion becomes translucent and the carrot begins to soften.
4. Add the chicken broth and kidney beans and bring to a simmer. Once the chicken is cooked, cut it into bite-size pieces. Add the kale and chicken to the pot, reduce the heat to medium low, and cook for 3 to 4 minutes. Discard the thyme sprig.

COOKING TIP: For a bit of added crunch and flavor, sprinkle on a few Italian-seasoned (containing parsley, oregano, and basil) bread crumbs to the chicken before you cook it. Be sure not to overcook the thighs or they will be too dry.

Per serving: Calories: 371; Fat: 13g; Sodium: 1,523mg; Carbohydrates: 33g; Fiber: 14g; Sugar: 5g; Protein: 30g

Kale and Apple Salad

Prep time: 15 minutes | Serves: 2

This is the salad that your family is going to want you to bring to the barbecue—even the non-lovers of kale will like it! It's packed with vitamins A, K, and C, all necessary for immune function. This can easily be gluten-free if you use gluten-free bread crumbs. Serve alone or with grilled chicken or fish.

For the dressing

¼ cup olive oil
2 tablespoons freshly squeezed lemon juice
1 small garlic clove, halved
1 teaspoon maple syrup, dark if you have it
¼ teaspoon salt

For the salad

2½ cups chopped kale
1 Honeycrisp apple, chopped
14 red grapes, halved
¼ cup sliced almonds
¼ cup plus 2 tablespoons grated Parmesan cheese (check label for vegetarian)
1 tablespoon bread crumbs

To make the dressing

1. In a bowl, combine the oil, lemon juice, garlic, maple syrup, and salt, and whisk to combine. Remove and discard the garlic halves just before using.

To make the salad

2. In a large bowl, combine the kale, apple, grapes, almonds, Parmesan cheese, bread crumbs, and dressing. Toss to coat.

VARIATION TIP: Use endive or sliced Bosc pears instead of the apple.

Per serving: Calories: 484; Fat: 37g; Sodium: 592mg; Carbohydrates: 34g; Fiber: 5g; Sugar: 30g; Protein: 9g

Mediterranean Quinoa and Kale Salad

Prep time: 15 minutes | Cook time: 10 minutes | Serves: 2

This is one of my favorite salads. The underlying flavors from the cucumber and feta cheese remind me of a classic Greek salad. This is great on its own but would also be lovely with a piece of grilled chicken breast with a little olive oil, salt, and pepper, or a piece of swordfish or tuna fish.

For the salad

1 cup water
½ cup quinoa, rinsed
2 cups chopped kale
8 cherry tomatoes, halved
½ cup chopped cucumber
8 kalamata olives, halved
½ teaspoon salt
¼ teaspoon freshly ground black pepper
¾ cup crumbled feta cheese

For the dressing

¼ cup olive oil
2 tablespoons red wine vinegar
½ teaspoon Dijon mustard
⅛ teaspoon salt
Freshly ground black pepper

To make the salad

1. In a 2-quart pot, bring the water and quinoa to a boil over high heat. Reduce the heat to low, cover, and simmer until the water has been absorbed and the quinoa is tender, about 10 minutes.
2. While the quinoa is cooking, in a large bowl, add the kale, tomatoes, cucumber, olives, salt, and pepper, and mix to combine.

To make the dressing

3. In a mason jar, combine the oil, red wine vinegar, mustard, salt, and pepper to taste. Shake well to incorporate.
4. Once the quinoa is finished cooking, fluff with a fork and add to the kale mixture along with the dressing and toss to combine. Top with the crumbled feta.

COOKING TIP: Make extra quinoa and use it in the Pecan-Cinnamon Breakfast Quinoa (page 30).

Per serving: Calories: 606; Fat: 46g; Sodium: 1,525mg; Carbohydrates: 34g; Fiber: 4g; Sugar: 5g; Protein: 15g

Spring Vegetable Quinoa Salad

Prep time: 15 minutes | Cook time: 15 minutes | Serves: 2

Inspired by a love for spring, this salad is packed with flavor, color, fiber, and protein. You can always change out the veggies for your personal favorites. If you want leftovers, double the recipe and pack it up for lunch the next day.

For the salad

2½ cups water, divided
½ cup quinoa, rinsed
½ cup shelled edamame
⅔ cup shredded or thinly sliced red cabbage
1 carrot, cut into matchsticks (about ½ cup)
½ red bell pepper, thinly sliced
⅓ cucumber, chopped (about ½ cup)
3 tablespoons chopped fresh cilantro

For the dressing

2 tablespoons rice wine vinegar
½ teaspoon tamari
¼ teaspoon sesame oil
1 scallion, white part only, sliced
1 teaspoon sesame seeds, for garnish

To make the salad

1. In a medium saucepan, bring 1 cup of water and the quinoa to a boil over high heat. Reduce the heat to low, cover, and simmer until the water has been absorbed and the quinoa is tender, about 10 minutes. Remove the pot from the heat and fluff with a fork.
2. In a small saucepan, bring the remaining 1½ cups of water to a boil and add the edamame. Cook for 3 minutes, drain, and let cool.
3. In a medium bowl, combine the red cabbage, carrot sticks, bell pepper, cucumber, and cilantro. Add the cooled quinoa and edamame and mix.

To make the dressing

4. In a separate small bowl, whisk the rice wine vinegar, tamari, sesame oil, and scallion. Pour the dressing over the quinoa mixture and stir to combine. Sprinkle the sesame seeds on top for garnish.

SUBSTITUTION TIP: If you don't have edamame on hand, use green peas or sugar snap peas.

Per serving: Calories: 262; Fat: 6g; Sodium: 126mg; Carbohydrates: 41g; Fiber: 8.5g; Sugar: 6g; Protein: 13g

Tuscan Chicken Sandwiches

Prep time: 5 minutes | Cook time: 15 minutes | Makes: 2 sandwiches

These chicken sandwiches are low in fat because they use chicken breast, but there's still plenty of flavor. Pesto brings that summertime feel, especially as it's combined with tomatoes. The sourdough bread helps bring the flavors together, but you can change it out for another that you prefer or have on hand. You may want to serve it with the Kale and Apple Salad (page 40).

- 2 (6- to 8-ounce) boneless, skinless chicken breasts
- 1 tablespoon olive oil
- ½ teaspoon salt
- Freshly ground black pepper
- ¼ cup Spinach and Basil Pesto (page 114)
- 4 slices sourdough bread
- 1 cup grated Havarti cheese
- 1 plum tomato, cut into 4 slices
- 1 tablespoon balsamic vinegar

1. Preheat an indoor or outdoor grill to medium heat.
2. Rub the chicken with the oil and season with the salt and pepper. Grill the chicken for 10 to 12 minutes or until an internal temperature of 165°F is reached.
3. Coat the chicken with the pesto and add a piece of chicken to each of two slices of the bread. Top with the cheese and tomato and drizzle 1½ teaspoons of balsamic vinegar over each. Cover with another slice of bread and halve.

COOKING TIP: After putting the pesto on the chicken and topping it with the cheese, you can heat the sandwich in the oven to melt the cheese if desired. If using a microwave, be careful not to cook too long and burn the cheese. Hold off on the tomato and vinegar until the cheese is melted.

Per serving (1 sandwich): Calories: 912; Fat: 47g; Sodium: 1,737mg; Carbohydrates: 55g; Fiber: 2.5g; Sugar: 6.5g; Protein: 65g

Grilled Eggplant Sandwiches

Prep time: 10 minutes | Cook time: 10 minutes | Makes: 2 sandwiches

Sandwiches always remind me of school lunches as a kid, but this sandwich is all grown-up and delicious. It's plant based yet filling, and the yogurt dressing adds a little tanginess, a perfect match for the tomato and eggplant.

- ¼ cup plain low-fat Greek yogurt
- 2 teaspoons freshly squeezed lemon juice
- ½ teaspoon dried oregano
- ¼ teaspoon salt
- ⅛ teaspoon minced garlic
- 10 ounces eggplant, peeled and cut into 8 to 10 thin slices
- ½ small red onion, cut into 4 slices
- ¼ cup olive oil
- 1 plum tomato, cut into 4 slices
- 4 slices bread, e.g., pita, sourdough, or focaccia

1. In a small bowl, mix the yogurt, lemon juice, oregano, salt, and garlic, and set aside, allowing the mixture to marinate while you prepare the vegetables.
2. Preheat an indoor or outdoor grill to medium heat.
3. Brush the eggplant and onion slices with oil and grill for 4 to 5 minutes on each side, until the onions and eggplant are softened. You can also toast the bread on the grill if desired. Toward the end of cooking, add the tomato slices and grill for only about 1 minute, being sure not to overcook. Remove all the vegetables from the grill.
4. Divide the grilled vegetables and layer the eggplant, onion, and tomato onto each of two bread slices. Spread the dressing onto the two top slices before assembling the sandwiches. Cut in half.

USE IT UP: If you have extra eggplant left over, you can cut it into pieces and roast it to use in other salads or as a side vegetable for dinner tonight. Try putting the extra eggplant to the Pasta with Veggie Spring Sauce (page 51) or the Veggie Pot Pies (page 53).

Per serving (1 sandwich): Calories: 542; Fat: 31g; Sodium: 736mg; Carbohydrates: 56g; Fiber: 6g; Sugar: 11g; Protein: 5g

Roasted Tomato and Portobello Sandwiches

Prep time: 5 minutes | Cook time: 10 minutes | Makes: 2 sandwiches

Mushrooms are low in calories and carbohydrates and contain a small amount of protein. The nutrients from tomatoes are more readily available when they are cooked slightly, so roasting them here means you get the full value of the lycopene, an antioxidant that fights off chronic diseases and cancer.

- 1 (4-ounce) portobello mushroom, sliced
- 1 large tomato, sliced (about 4 slices)
- Olive oil, for roasting
- 1 teaspoon chopped fresh thyme
- ¼ teaspoon salt
- ¼ teaspoon freshly ground black pepper
- ⅓ cup crumbled goat cheese
- ½ cup arugula
- ½ teaspoon freshly squeezed lemon juice
- 2 ciabatta rolls, halved
- ¼ teaspoon grated Parmesan cheese (check label for vegetarian)
- 6 pitted black olives

1. Preheat the oven to 400°F.
2. On a baking sheet, place the mushroom and tomato slices and drizzle with oil. Season with the thyme, salt, and pepper. Bake for about 6 minutes or until the tomatoes soften but are not mushy.
3. Add the goat cheese on top of the tomatoes and bake for another 1 minute. Remove from the oven.
4. Toss the arugula with the lemon juice. Divide the mushrooms and tomatoes between the two rolls and top with the Parmesan cheese, arugula, and olives. Season with salt and pepper before adding the top of the roll.

SUBSTITUTION TIP: To make this vegan, omit the goat cheese and Parmesan.

Per serving (1 sandwich): Calories: 319; Fat: 12g; Sodium: 925mg; Carbohydrates: 41g; Fiber: 4.5g; Sugar: 5g; Protein: 11g

Vegan Tomato Bisque

Prep time: 10 minutes | Cook time: 10 minutes | Serves: 2

Most tomato bisques are made using heavy whipping cream. To make this classic soup vegan, I use cashew cream instead. Cashew milk is quite easy to make at home from raw cashews, and you can use it in place of cream in any recipe.

For the cashew cream

1 cup water
½ cup raw unsalted cashews
1 tablespoon freshly squeezed lemon juice
1 teaspoon salt
½ teaspoon freshly ground black pepper

For the soup

1 tablespoon olive oil
2 tablespoons finely diced shallot
1 garlic clove, minced
1 (28-ounce) can whole tomatoes
1 teaspoon chopped fresh thyme, plus more for garnish
Freshly ground black pepper

To make the cashew cream

1. In a blender or food processor, combine the water, cashews, lemon juice, salt, and pepper. Blend until smooth. Set aside.

To make the soup

2. In a 4-quart saucepan, heat the oil over medium heat and cook the shallot and garlic until fragrant, about 1 minute. Add the tomatoes and their juices and stir while carefully smashing the tomatoes with the back of the spoon. Stir in the thyme, season with pepper, and bring to a simmer.
3. Once simmering, remove from the heat and add half the cashew cream. Blend using an immersion blender, regular blender, or potato masher.
4. Divide the soup into two bowls and garnish with a swirl of the remaining cashew cream and fresh thyme.

VARIATION TIP: You can still enjoy this without the cream. It will be less creamy, but you can continue to cook the soup after blending to reduce it and thicken it up.

Per serving: Calories: 313; Fat: 19g; Sodium: 1,765mg; Carbohydrates: 24g; Fiber: 4.5g; Sugar: 13g; Protein: 9g

Coconut Chicken Soup

Prep time: 10 minutes | Cook time: 20 minutes | Serves: 2

This is a refreshing soup any time of the year. The coconut milk helps bring all the flavors together while still allowing the brothy flavor to come through. The cilantro and mushrooms help with detoxing and are anti-inflammatory. You can omit the chicken and use vegetable broth for a vegetarian variation of the soup.

- 1 tablespoon olive oil
- ½ cup chopped carrot
- ½ cup chopped onion
- ½ cup chopped celery
- 12 ounces boneless, skinless chicken breast, cubed
- ½ cup chopped mushrooms
- 1 bay leaf
- ½ teaspoon ground ginger
- 2 cups low-sodium chicken broth
- ⅔ cup canned light coconut milk
- 2 tablespoons chopped fresh cilantro
- 1½ teaspoons freshly squeezed lime juice
- ⅛ teaspoon red pepper flakes
- ½ teaspoon salt
- ¼ teaspoon freshly ground black pepper

1. In a 4-quart pot, heat the oil over medium heat and sauté the carrot, onion, and celery. When the onion begins to soften, add the chicken and cook for about 5 minutes or until the chicken turns white on the outside.
2. Add the mushrooms, bay leaf, and ginger. Continue to sauté for another 1 minute, giving it a stir to combine the ingredients. Add the broth and bring to a boil. Reduce the heat to low and simmer for another 10 minutes or until the internal temperature of the chicken is 165°F and the chicken is cooked through.
3. Remove and discard the bay leaf. Add the coconut milk and heat through, then add the cilantro, lime juice, and red pepper flakes. Season with the salt and pepper. Simmer for 1 more minute, then serve.

COOKING TIP: Try to have the chicken pieces about the same thickness so the cooking time is even. If you have leftover chicken from another dish, you can shred or cube it and reduce the cooking time when you add the broth to 5 minutes.

SUBSTITUTION TIP: If you have fresh ginger, you can substitute it for the ground ginger, using 1 teaspoon of minced fresh ginger.

Per serving: Calories: 367; Fat: 15g; Sodium: 798mg; Carbohydrates: 14g; Fiber: 2.5g; Sugar: 6g; Protein: 42g

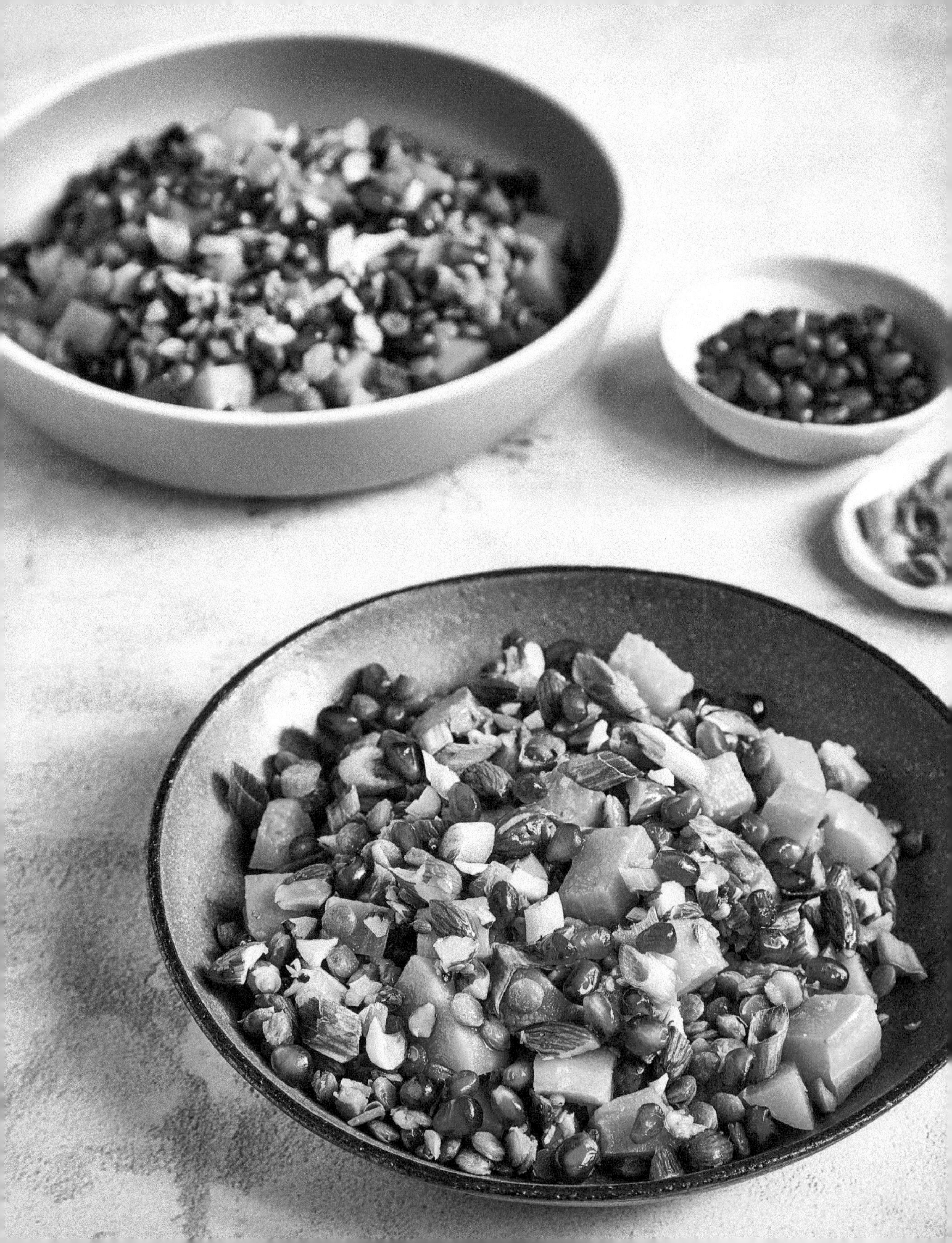

CHAPTER FOUR

Vegan and Vegetarian

Spaghetti Squash with Pesto

Prep time: 15 minutes | Cook time: 20 minutes | Serves: 2

Gluten-Free, Vegetarian

Spaghetti squash can make any pasta dish more fun. The beta carotene in the squash gives it the orangish color, and it's an antioxidant that helps fight off cancer and cell damage.

- 1 (3-pound) spaghetti squash
- 6 ounces cherry tomatoes, halved
- 1 teaspoon olive oil
- 1 tablespoon pumpkin seeds
- ⅓ cup Spinach and Basil Pesto (page 114)
- Grated Parmesan cheese, for garnish (check label for vegetarian)

1. Preheat the oven to 425°F.
2. Using a knife, cut slits in the squash along the midline lengthwise. Poke the squash in a few places with a fork or paring knife to allow steam to escape when cooking.
3. Put the squash in the microwave and cook for 5 minutes. Carefully take it out (it will be very hot) and cut it in half where you put the slits on the side. Remove the seeds.
4. Put one squash half, cut-side down, into a microwaveable baking dish. Add enough water so that it's about 1 inch deep. Microwave for another 5 minutes. Repeat the process with the other squash half.
5. On a baking sheet, toss the tomatoes with the oil and put in the oven for 7 to 8 minutes, making sure they remain firm.
6. While the tomatoes are cooking, in a small sauté pan, toast the pumpkin seeds over low heat until fragrant.
7. Once both halves of the squash are cooked, remove from the baking dish and, using a fork, scrape the strands of squash away from the skin. Put the squash in a medium bowl.
8. Toss the squash with the pesto and top with the pumpkin seeds and tomatoes. Garnish with the Parmesan cheese and serve.

VARIATION TIP: Add tofu: Bake the tofu for 15 to 18 minutes, until golden.

Per serving (without garnish): Calories: 444; Fat: 32g; Sodium: 301mg; Carbohydrates: 38g; Fiber: 9g; Sugar: 15g; Protein: 7g

Pasta with Veggie Spring Sauce

Prep time: 15 minutes | Cook time: 30 minutes | Serves: 2

I love this meal because it is low calorie, high fiber, and dense in nutrients. It is packed with B vitamins and vitamin C, and even though it's pasta, it is still guilt-free. It would go well with sautéed broccoli rabe to finish it off.

- 8 cups water
- 4 ounces bow tie pasta
- ⅔ cup coarsely chopped onion
- ⅔ cup coarsely chopped carrot
- ⅔ cup coarsely chopped eggplant
- ½ cup coarsely chopped celery
- ¼ cup chopped mushrooms
- 3 tablespoons olive oil
- 3 tablespoons white wine (optional)
- 1¼ cups tomato puree
- 2 tablespoons chopped fresh basil
- 1 tablespoon chopped fresh parsley
- ¾ teaspoon salt
- ¼ teaspoon freshly ground black pepper
- Grated Parmesan cheese, for garnish (check label for vegetarian)

1. Fill a 4-quart pot with the water and bring to a boil. Add the pasta and cook for about 8 minutes or until al dente.
2. Place the onion, carrot, eggplant, celery, and mushrooms in a food processor and pulse the vegetables until they are in small, uniform pieces, being careful not to puree them.
3. In a 2-quart pot, heat the oil over medium heat. Add the chopped vegetables and cook for about 10 minutes, until slightly softened. Add the white wine (if using) and cook for another 2 minutes.
4. Add the tomato puree, basil, parsley, salt, and pepper, and continue to cook for about 10 minutes, until the sauce is heated through and the flavors are combined.
5. Pour the sauce over the cooked noodles. Garnish with the Parmesan cheese to serve.

SUBSTITUTION TIP: If you do not have basil, use some Spinach and Basil Pesto (page 114) instead.

Per serving (without garnish): Calories: 501; Fat: 22g; Sodium: 1,242mg; Carbohydrates: 68g; Fiber: 8.5g; Sugar: 15g; Protein: 11g

Zesty Hotcakes with Lemon-Yogurt Sauce

Prep time: 10 minutes | Cook time: 10 minutes | Makes: 4 hotcakes

Quick, Gluten-Free, Vegetarian

These hotcakes are packed with flavor from the spice mix of thyme, paprika, and cumin. They provide a bit of protein and iron from the spinach. You can change out the spinach for any leafy green. Serve these with a salad.

For the hotcakes

1½ cups almond flour
¼ teaspoon salt
⅛ teaspoon dried thyme
⅛ teaspoon paprika
⅛ teaspoon ground cumin
½ cup water
5 thin red onion slices, almost shaved
1 cup packed baby spinach, leaves halved
2 tablespoons olive oil
Freshly ground black pepper

For the sauce

¼ cup plain low-fat Greek yogurt
½ teaspoon freshly squeezed lemon juice
¼ teaspoon sea salt
¼ teaspoon red pepper flakes

To make the hotcakes

1. In a medium bowl, combine the almond flour, salt, thyme, paprika, and cumin. Slowly stir in the water until the consistency is thinner than pancake batter but not as thin as water. (You may not need all the water.) Allow the batter to sit for 1 to 2 minutes.
2. Put the onion slices and spinach in the batter and mix.
3. In a 10-inch nonstick skillet or sauté pan, heat the oil over medium to high heat. Divide the batter into quarters, using a large spoon, along with your hand to pick up some of the vegetables and place them in the heated pan.
4. Allow the hotcakes to cook on one side for 3 minutes or until golden in color; turn over and continue cooking on the other side.

To make the sauce

5. In a small bowl, whisk together the yogurt, lemon juice, salt, and red pepper flakes. Divide the hotcakes between two plates and drizzle the yogurt sauce over each.

SUBSTITUTION TIP: Kale would be a great alternative to spinach.

Per serving (2 hotcakes): Calories: 458; Fat: 36g; Sodium: 621mg; Carbohydrates: 17g; Fiber: 10g; Sugar: 4.5g; Protein: 19g

Veggie Pot Pies

Prep time: 10 minutes | Cook time: 20 minutes | Serves: 2

You will never miss the meat in this vegetarian version of pot pie. I highly recommend making a double batch and storing the other half in your freezer for later. This version contains lentils, which are heart healthy because they contain fiber, folic acid, and potassium. Serve with a salad.

- 1 pound white potatoes, peeled and quartered
- 1 tablespoon olive oil
- ½ cup chopped onion
- 1 cup frozen peas and carrots
- 1 cup canned lentils, rinsed
- ½ cup chopped cremini or white button mushrooms
- 1 tablespoon all-purpose flour
- 1¼ cups vegetable broth
- ¼ cup reduced-fat milk
- 1 tablespoon butter
- 1 teaspoon salt
- ¼ teaspoon freshly ground black pepper
- ¼ cup grated Cheddar cheese

1. In a large pot, cover the potatoes with water and bring to a boil. Cook for about 10 minutes or until the potatoes are fork-tender.
2. Preheat the broiler.
3. While the potatoes are cooking, in a skillet, heat the oil over medium heat. Add the onion and sauté for 4 to 5 minutes, until soft.
4. Add the peas and carrots and cook for 1 minute. Add the lentils and mushrooms and stir until heated through.
5. Add the flour and stir to combine. Pour in the broth, bring to a boil, then lower the heat and simmer until the mixture thickens.
6. Once the potatoes are cooked, drain them and set aside. Add the milk and butter to the pot and stir to warm through, then place the potatoes back in the pot and mash until smooth. Season with the salt and pepper.
7. Divide the vegetable mixture into two oven-safe serving dishes and top with the mashed potatoes. Sprinkle the cheese on top and place under the broiler for about 3 minutes or until the cheese is melted.

USE IT UP: Leftover lentils can be used in salads or grain bowls, or even in the Weekend Breakfast Burrito (page 27).

Per serving: Calories: 463; Fat: 12g; Sodium: 1,529mg; Carbohydrates: 72g; Fiber: 18g; Sugar: 9.5g; Protein: 20g

Black-and-White Burgers

Prep time: 15 minutes | Cook time: 10 minutes
Makes: 2 (5-ounce) burgers

These burgers have a wonderfully smooth texture due to the creaminess of the white beans, and they are packed with fiber and protein. The flaxseed adds a heart-healthy component, and oatmeal is great for lowering cholesterol. Serve on buns with fresh tomato slices or over a salad.

- 1 tablespoon olive oil, divided
- 2 tablespoons chopped shallot
- 1½ ounces white button mushrooms, chopped
- ¼ teaspoon ground cumin
- ½ cup rolled oats
- ½ cup canned navy beans, drained and rinsed
- ½ cup canned black beans, drained and rinsed
- ¼ cup plain bread crumbs (confirm dairy-free if needed)
- 1 large egg
- 1 teaspoon ground flaxseed
- ¼ teaspoon salt

1. In a skillet or sauté pan, heat ½ tablespoon of oil over medium heat, and sauté the shallot and mushrooms until the shallot is translucent and the mushrooms are soft, about 1 minute. Add the cumin, cook until fragrant, and remove from the heat.
2. In a food processor, pulse the oats. Add the navy beans, black beans, bread crumbs, egg, flaxseed, salt, and the cooked shallot and mushroom mix, and blend for 4 minutes, scraping down the sides as needed to ensure that everything is mixed thoroughly.
3. Divide the mixture in half and form into two patties.
4. Heat the remaining ½ tablespoon of oil in the same pan. Cook the burgers for 4 minutes on each side, until browned, and serve.

USE IT UP: Leftover beans can be frozen, or double the recipe and make extra burgers for another day. The burgers freeze well. Take them out at the last minute and place them in a 400°F oven.

Per serving (1 burger): Calories: 278; Fat: 5g; Sodium: 869mg; Carbohydrates: 44g; Fiber: 11g; Sugar: 3g; Protein: 15g

Rice Noodle and Vegetable Bowls

Prep time: 10 minutes | Cook time: 10 minutes | Serves: 2

Quick, Gluten-Free, Vegan

This noodle bowl is my version of cozy food. The mushrooms not only provide the umami flavor but also boost your immune system, and they are a rich source of potassium, which can potentially lower blood pressure. Spinach is rich in vitamins A, C, and K, and it's perfect for improving skin texture. If you want to spice it up, top with a bit of sriracha.

- 4 ounces rice noodles
- 1½ tablespoons olive oil
- 1 small carrot, cut into matchsticks
- 5 ounces shiitake mushrooms, sliced
- ½ cup frozen shelled edamame
- 3 scallions, both white and green parts, sliced
- 2 tablespoons chickpea miso
- 1 teaspoon grated fresh ginger
- 3 cups vegetable broth
- 2 cups fresh spinach
- 2 tablespoons sesame oil
- 1 teaspoon salt
- ½ teaspoon freshly ground black pepper

1. Fill a 4-quart pot with water and bring to a boil. Once the water comes to a boil, add the rice noodles and cook for 5 minutes or until tender. Drain and divide them between two bowls.
2. In another pot, heat the oil over medium heat. Add the carrot. Cook for 1 minute, then add the mushrooms, edamame, and scallions. Sauté until the mixture is soft, 1 to 2 minutes.
3. Add the miso paste and ginger to the skillet and stir, cooking for about 30 seconds.
4. Add the vegetable broth and simmer for 2 minutes. Add the spinach and cook until it wilts. Remove from the heat, stir in the sesame oil, and season with the salt and pepper.
5. Divide the vegetable mixture between the bowls with the rice noodles, and serve.

SUBSTITUTION TIP: I used chickpea miso, but you can also use white miso without changing the flavor.

Per serving: Calories: 576; Fat: 28g; Sodium: 1,939mg; Carbohydrates: 70g; Fiber: 11g; Sugar: 7.5g; Protein: 15g

Chickpea Grain Bowls with Avocado and Feta

Prep time: 15 minutes | Cook time: 25 minutes | Serves: 2

These bowls are packed with so much flavor that they don't need much dressing or sauce. Try just a little olive or avocado oil and vinegar. Tahini Dressing (page 116) would be a delicious option, too.

- 1½ cups water
- ½ cup pearled barley
- 1 bay leaf
- 6 ounces eggplant, peeled and cubed
- 2 tablespoons olive oil, divided
- 2 ounces shiitake mushrooms, sliced
- 2 cups coarsely chopped mixed greens
- 1 cup canned chickpeas, drained and rinsed
- 1 avocado, cubed
- ½ cup crumbled feta cheese
- 1 tablespoon pistachios, coarsely chopped
- 2 teaspoons sliced scallions, white part only, sliced on an angle

1. Preheat the oven to 400°F. Line a baking sheet with parchment paper.
2. In a 2-quart pot, bring the water to a boil. Add the barley and bay leaf. Return to a boil, then reduce the heat, cover, and simmer until tender, 20 to 23 minutes. Remove and discard the bay leaf.
3. In a large bowl, drizzle the eggplant with 1½ tablespoons of oil. Toss and place on the prepared baking sheet and cook for 20 minutes or until golden brown.
4. In a small nonstick pan, heat the remaining ½ tablespoon of oil and sauté the mushrooms for about 5 minutes, until softened.
5. Once the eggplant, mushrooms, and barley are cooked, place a portion of each into two serving bowls.
6. In a separate large bowl, combine the greens, chickpeas, avocado, feta cheese, pistachios, and scallions and toss to combine. Divide this mixture and add to the bowls with the barley mixture. Add any dressing before serving.

SUBSTITUTION TIP: If barley is not for you, try farro instead. To make this recipe gluten-free, swap quinoa or brown rice for the barley.

Per serving: Calories: 673; Fat: 36g; Sodium: 555mg; Carbohydrates: 74g; Fiber: 22g; Sugar: 9g; Protein: 20g

Ultimate Falafel Burgers

Prep time: 15 minutes, plus 8 to 12 hours to soak overnight
Cook time: 10 minutes | Makes: 2 burgers

This recipe takes a bit of planning, as you will need to soak the chickpeas overnight, but it is worth it. Canned chickpeas will not create the correct falafel texture, so be sure to use dry.

- ½ cup chickpeas, soaked overnight
- ½ cup fresh parsley
- ½ cup fresh cilantro
- ¼ onion, peeled
- 1 garlic clove, peeled
- ½ teaspoon ground cumin
- ½ teaspoon ground coriander
- ½ teaspoon salt
- ¼ cup finely grated carrot
- 2 tablespoons chickpea flour
- ¼ teaspoon baking powder
- 2 teaspoons avocado oil, divided
- 4 slices bread or 2 burger buns
- Carrot and Cucumber Yogurt Sauce (page 121)

1. In a food processor, combine the chickpeas, parsley, cilantro, onion, garlic, cumin, coriander, and salt. Pulse until combined, scraping down the sides as needed.
2. Pour the mixture into a bowl and add the carrot, flour, and baking powder, and mix to combine. Divide the mixture and shape it into two patties.
3. In a skillet or sauté pan, heat 1 teaspoon of oil over medium heat. Add the patties and cook for 4 to 5 minutes on each side or until crispy and golden brown. Add the remaining 1 teaspoon of oil as needed.
4. Assemble the burgers on bread and top each with half of the yogurt sauce (tzatziki).

COOKING TIP: Instead of panfrying, you can bake the falafel in the oven at 375°F for 20 minutes, flipping them halfway through.

Per serving (1 burger): Calories: 565; Fat: 14g; Sodium: 1,028mg; Carbohydrates: 76g; Fiber: 14g; Sugar: 17g; Protein: 34g

Spiced Lentils with Butternut Squash

Prep time: 10 minutes | Cook time: 25 minutes | Serves: 2

Gluten-Free, Vegan

Lentils are packed full of fiber and protein, making them a great plant-based protein alternative. This recipe is bursting with flavor, which comes from infusing the oil with aromatics.

- 2 cups finely cubed butternut squash
- ¼ cup olive oil, plus 1 teaspoon
- ¼ teaspoon salt, plus more for seasoning
- ¼ teaspoon freshly ground black pepper
- 2 scallions, both white and green parts, sliced and divided
- 2 garlic cloves, smashed
- 1 (3-inch) lemon peel
- 2 thyme sprigs
- ¼ cup whole almonds, coarsely chopped
- ¼ teaspoon coriander seeds
- ⅛ teaspoon red pepper flakes
- 2 tablespoons freshly squeezed lemon juice
- 1 cup canned lentils, drained and rinsed
- Pomegranate arils, for serving (optional)

1. Preheat the oven to 425°F.
2. On a baking sheet, arrange the butternut squash and toss with 1 teaspoon of oil, the salt, and pepper. Roast for 15 to 20 minutes, until the squash is cooked through.
3. In a small skillet or sauté pan, heat the remaining ¼ cup of oil over medium heat and add the white part of the scallions, garlic, lemon peel, and thyme sprigs. Cook over medium-low heat until the garlic is slightly browned and the lemon peel begins to curl.
4. Add the almonds and cook for 3 to 4 minutes, until fragrant.

5. Remove from the heat and add the coriander seeds and red pepper flakes. Stir to combine and let cool slightly.
6. Strain the oil into a bowl using either a fine mesh strainer or the back of a large spoon. Scatter the almond mixture onto a plate and pick out the garlic cloves, thyme sprigs, and lemon peel. Lightly season the almonds with salt and set aside.
7. Add the lemon juice to the oil and whisk.
8. Combine the lentils and butternut squash in a medium bowl. Pour in the dressing and add the almonds. Stir to combine. Season with salt and pepper. Divide between two bowls and top with the scallion greens and pomegranate arils (if using) to serve.

Per serving: Calories: 594; Fat: 37g; Sodium: 300mg; Carbohydrates: 52g; Fiber: 14g; Sugar: 4.5g; Protein: 18g

Roasted Ruby Cabbage

Prep time: 10 minutes | Cook time: 35 minutes | Serves: 2

Gluten-Free, Vegan

My favorite way to prepare red cabbage is to roast it as featured in this recipe. I also add nuts and sweet and tangy dried cranberries, as well as some Granny Smith apple. The balsamic vinegar rounds out the flavors and creates a dish you will want to make time and time again.

- 4 cups thinly sliced red cabbage
- 1 tablespoon olive oil
- ½ teaspoon garlic powder
- ½ teaspoon paprika
- ¼ teaspoon salt
- Pinch freshly ground black pepper
- ⅓ cup raw pecan halves
- ½ cup diced Granny Smith apple
- ¼ cup unsweetened or juice-sweetened dried cranberries
- 1 teaspoon balsamic vinegar

1. Preheat the oven to 425°F.
2. Put the cabbage on a parchment-lined baking sheet.
3. Drizzle with the oil and season with the garlic powder, paprika, salt, and pepper. Mix to combine and roast for 30 to 35 minutes, until the cabbage is light brown and slightly crispy.
4. While the cabbage is roasting, in a small skillet, toast the pecans over medium-low heat for 1 to 2 minutes, until fragrant and slightly darker in color. Remove from the heat, coarsely chop, and set aside.
5. Once cooked, transfer the cabbage to a large bowl and add the apple, pecans, and cranberries, and drizzle with the balsamic vinegar. Toss to combine and serve.

VARIATION TIP: Another variation on the spices is to swap the same amount of curry powder for the paprika and garlic powder.

Per serving: Calories: 284; Fat: 19g; Sodium: 329mg; Carbohydrates: 29g; Fiber: 6g; Sugar: 19g; Protein: 3g

Rice and Beans

Prep time: 10 minutes | Cook time: 20 minutes | Serves: 2

Rice and beans make a complete protein, which means you get all the essential amino acids. Amino acids are building blocks and help tissue repair and nutrient absorption. Try serving this with a side of sautéed vegetables such as spinach.

- 2 tablespoons avocado oil
- ½ medium sweet onion, chopped
- ½ cup chopped green bell pepper
- ¼ cup chopped red bell pepper
- 1 jalapeño pepper, chopped
- 1 garlic clove, minced
- ¼ teaspoon dried thyme
- ¼ teaspoon fresh thyme
- ¼ teaspoon cayenne pepper
- ¼ teaspoon red pepper flakes
- 1 cup canned red beans, drained and rinsed
- 3 ripe plum tomatoes (very ripe), diced
- 1 cup vegetable broth
- ½ cup basmati rice or brown rice
- ¼ cup water
- ⅛ teaspoon salt
- Freshly ground black pepper
- 1 scallion, both white and green parts, sliced, for garnish

1. In a 4-quart pot, heat the oil over medium heat. Add the onion, bell peppers, jalapeño, and garlic, and sauté for 2 to 3 minutes, until tender.
2. Add the dry and fresh thyme, cayenne pepper, and red pepper flakes, and mix well.
3. Add the beans and heat through, about 1 minute. Add the tomatoes, vegetable broth, rice, and water, and bring to a boil. Cover, reduce the heat to low, stirring occasionally, and cook for 15 minutes or until the rice is cooked.
4. Add the salt and season with pepper to taste. Garnish with the scallion slices.

SUBSTITUTION TIP: If you have dried thyme, you can use it instead of fresh.

Per serving: Calories: 476; Fat: 14g; Sodium: 652mg; Carbohydrates: 75g; Fiber: 11g; Sugar: 12g; Protein: 13g

Lentil-Quinoa Stir-Fry

Prep time: 10 minutes | Cook time: 15 minutes | Serves: 2

Quick, Gluten-Free, Vegan

This quinoa stir-fry is a cleaner replacement for your typical fried rice. It has protein and fiber thanks to the quinoa and lentils. Served over the spinach, it gets a dose of vitamin K and more fiber as well as some B vitamins. Using coconut aminos keeps it soy- and gluten-free.

- 1½ cups water
- ⅔ cup quinoa, rinsed
- ½ tablespoon olive oil
- ½ cup chopped onion
- ½ cup chopped green bell pepper
- ½ cup chopped red bell pepper
- ¼ cup plus 1 tablespoon chopped mushrooms
- ½ cup cooked lentils
- 2 teaspoons walnuts, chopped
- 2 cups chopped spinach
- 1½ tablespoons sesame oil
- 1 tablespoon coconut aminos or tamari

1. In a 2-quart pot, bring the water and quinoa to a boil over high heat. Reduce the heat to low, cover, and simmer until the water has been absorbed and the quinoa is tender, about 10 minutes.
2. In a nonstick skillet or sauté pan, heat the oil over medium heat and sauté the onion and bell peppers for about 2 minutes, until slightly soft. Add the mushrooms and sauté for another 30 seconds.
3. Add the lentils and walnuts, stirring to combine and heat through, about 30 seconds.
4. Add the quinoa, spinach, sesame oil, and coconut aminos, stirring to combine all the ingredients.
5. Serve warm.

USE IT UP: This is the perfect dish to use up any leftover quinoa you may have in the refrigerator.

Per serving: Calories: 457; Fat: 19g; Sodium: 280mg; Carbohydrates: 58g; Fiber: 11g; Sugar: 8g; Protein: 15g

Eggplant and Zucchini Bake

Prep time: 15 minutes | Cook time: 30 minutes | Serves: 2

Gluten-Free, Vegetarian

This bake is flavorful and will make you feel like you're having lasagna. Low in carbohydrates and high in fiber, this lasagna remake will provide your body with antioxidants, minerals, and vitamins. Serve with Kale and Apple Salad (page 40).

- 8 ounces eggplant, peeled and cut lengthwise into thin strips (5 or 6 slices)
- 8 ounces zucchini, peeled and cut lengthwise into thin strips (5 or 6 slices)
- 1½ tablespoons olive oil
- 3 cups tomato sauce
- 1 tablespoon Italian seasoning
- ½ teaspoon salt
- ¼ teaspoon freshly ground black pepper
- 1 small red onion, thinly sliced
- 5 ounces button mushrooms, sliced
- 1 cup grated Parmesan cheese, divided (check label for vegetarian)

1. Preheat the oven to 425°F.
2. Put the eggplant and zucchini on a baking sheet and brush with the oil. Roast for about 6 minutes, until the eggplant is starting to soften.
3. In a small bowl, combine the tomato sauce, Italian seasoning, salt, and pepper, and stir.
4. In an 8-by-8-inch baking dish, pour just enough of the sauce mixture on the bottom to cover. Place a layer of roasted eggplant on top of the sauce and top with some of the onion slices, mushrooms, and zucchini.
5. Top with more sauce and sprinkle with ½ cup of cheese. Repeat the layering, starting with the eggplant, mushrooms, and onions and finishing the top layer with the zucchini and red sauce, topped with the remaining ½ cup of cheese.
6. Bake for 20 minutes or until the cheese is browning.

SUBSTITUTION TIP: If you make your own tomato sauce, feel free to use that instead of the tomato sauce in the recipe. And feel free to use any of your favorite mushrooms or a sweet onion. Use a vegan cheese instead of Parmesan if you want to make the dish vegan.

Per serving: Calories: 452; Fat: 19g; Sodium: 1,379mg; Carbohydrates: 59g; Fiber: 11g; Sugar: 27g; Protein: 12g

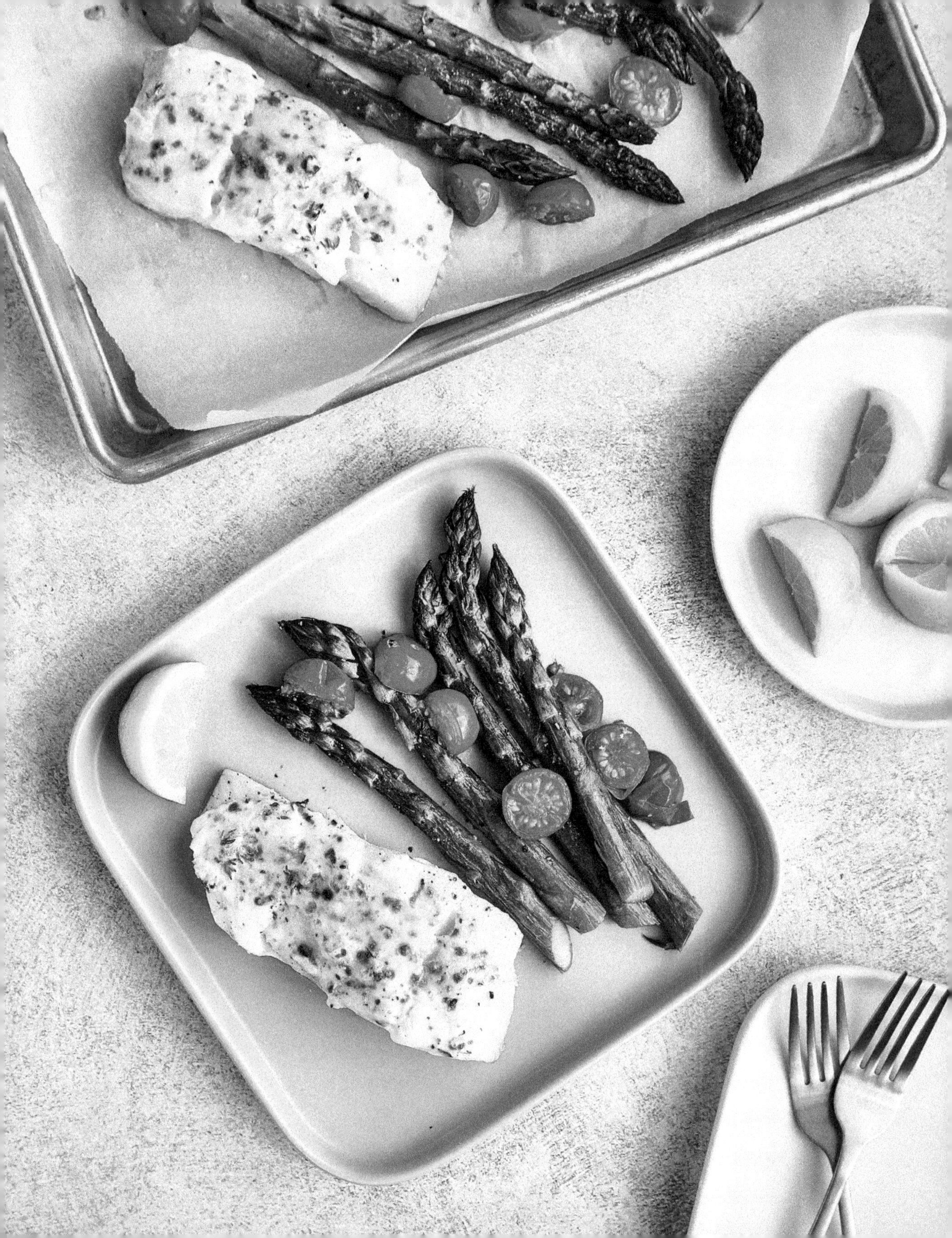

CHAPTER FIVE

Fish and Seafood

Sole Florentine

Prep time: 5 minutes | Cook time: 10 minute | Serves: 2

This is my version of this classic seafood dish. It requires minimal prep and is ready in under 20 minutes. Plate the fish over a bed of fresh baby spinach or serve with a side of rice. You can always feel like it's a special occasion with this clean and easy meal.

- 2 (6-ounce) sole fillets
- ½ teaspoon salt, plus more for seasoning
- ½ teaspoon freshly ground black pepper, plus more for seasoning
- 2 tablespoons bread crumbs (confirm dairy-free if needed)
- 1½ tablespoons freshly squeezed lemon juice
- 2 cups baby spinach
- 2 tablespoons water
- 1 lemon, cut into 4 wedges, for serving

1. Preheat the oven to 375°F. Line a baking sheet with parchment paper.
2. Season both sides of the fish with the salt and pepper and place on the prepared baking sheet. Sprinkle the bread crumbs on top and evenly cover with the lemon juice.
3. Bake until the fish is opaque or has an internal temperature of 145°F, about 10 minutes.
4. In a small skillet or sauté pan, heat the spinach and water over medium-low heat. Season with salt and pepper and cook until the spinach is wilted.
5. Divide the spinach between two plates and place the fish fillets on top. Serve with the lemon wedges.

SUBSTITUTION TIP: You can substitute red snapper or another white fish for the sole.

Per serving: Calories: 143; Fat: 3g; Sodium: 1,088mg; Carbohydrates: 8g; Fiber: 2g; Sugar: 1g; Protein: 20g

Quick Marinated Salmon

Prep time: 15 minutes | Cook time: 10 minutes | Serves: 2

Quick, Dairy-Free, Gluten-Free

This recipe is loaded with docosahexaenoic acid (DHA), an omega-3 fatty acid important for brain health, and ginger, which fights inflammation in the body. Best of all, it is simple and delicious. Serve the fillets with some steamed bok choy or a simple salad with olive oil and vinegar on the side.

¼ cup pineapple juice
2 tablespoons coconut aminos
1 tablespoon olive oil
1 teaspoon chopped scallions, both white and green parts
¾ teaspoon ground ginger
⅛ teaspoon hot sauce
2 (7-ounce) salmon fillets
1 tablespoon chopped fresh parsley
Lemon slices, for garnish (optional)

1. Preheat the oven to 350°F. Line a baking sheet with parchment paper.
2. In a medium bowl, mix the pineapple juice, coconut aminos, oil, scallions, ginger, and hot sauce.
3. Add the salmon fillets and coat well with the marinade. Marinate for 5 minutes or up to 12 hours.
4. Drain the marinade and put the fillets on the prepared baking sheet. Bake for 8 to 10 minutes or until firm.
5. Sprinkle with the parsley. Place the lemon slices (if using) on the side for garnish.

SUBSTITUTION TIP: You can use fresh ginger if you have it. To cut down on waste, look for a small can of pineapple juice instead of a larger bottle.

Per serving: Calories: 413; Fat: 21g; Sodium: 379mg; Carbohydrates: 7g; Fiber: 0g; Sugar: 6g; Protein: 45g

Quick

Happy Crab Cakes

Prep time: 10 minutes | Cook time: 10 minutes
Makes: 4 (3-ounce) crab cakes

I call these crab cakes "happy" because they are loaded with crab meat, and who doesn't love crab cakes? Crab meat is low in calories but high in vitamins and omega-3 fatty acids. It is also rich in zinc, which contributes to a strong immune system.

---

12 ounces crab meat
½ cup plain low-fat Greek yogurt
2 tablespoons chopped red bell pepper
2 tablespoons sliced scallions
⅔ cup bread crumbs, plus 1 tablespoon
½ teaspoon salt
¼ teaspoon freshly ground black pepper
2 tablespoons olive oil, plus more as needed
Lemon wedges, for serving

1. Squeeze out any excess water from the crab meat and pick out any shell bits.
2. Place the crab meat in a large bowl and add the yogurt, bell pepper, scallions, 1 tablespoon of bread crumbs, salt, and pepper. Stir to combine well.
3. Form the mixture into four equal patties. Spread the remaining ⅔ cup of bread crumbs on a plate and dip in each patty, coating both sides with bread crumbs.
4. In a 10-inch nonstick skillet or sauté pan, heat 2 tablespoons of oil over medium heat and swirl to coat the pan. Once hot, put the crab cakes in the pan and cook until they are golden on the bottom, 4 to 5 minutes. (You may need to add a little more oil here if the pan becomes too dry.) Turn the cakes over and continue cooking for another 4 to 5 minutes.
5. Serve hot with the lemon wedges.

VARIATION TIP: Pair with the Bell Pepper and Chickpea Salad (page 37) for a refreshing meal.

Per serving (2 crab cakes): Calories: 440; Fat: 18g; Sodium: 1,626mg; Carbohydrates: 31g; Fiber: 3.5g; Sugar: 5.5g; Protein: 39g

Veggie Scallop Bowls

Prep time: 15 minutes | Cook time: 20 minutes | Serves: 2

These scallop bowls are packed with protein from both the quinoa and the scallops. The pickled onions are tasty and, better yet, gut friendly. The sweet potato contains vitamin A for vision health and fiber for gut health.

- ½ cup thinly sliced red onion
- 2 tablespoons apple cider vinegar
- 1 tablespoon honey
- 1¼ cups water, divided
- ½ cup quinoa, rinsed
- 1 sweet potato
- 1 tablespoon olive oil
- 8 ounces sea scallops
- 1 tablespoon freshly squeezed lemon juice
- 2 cups spinach
- 1 cup canned chickpeas, rinsed and drained
- 4 tablespoons Tahini Dressing (page 116)
- Lemon wedge, for garnish

1. In a small bowl, put the onion, vinegar, and honey, and stir to combine. Set aside while you prepare the rest of the meal, stirring occasionally.
2. In a 2-quart pot, bring 1 cup of water and the quinoa to a boil over high heat. Reduce the heat to low, cover, and simmer until the water has been absorbed and the quinoa is tender, about 10 minutes. Remove the pot from the heat and fluff the quinoa with a fork.
3. Microwave the sweet potato on high for 4 to 5 minutes.
4. In a nonstick skillet or sauté pan, heat the oil over medium heat. Add the scallops and cook for about 2 minutes or until golden brown on one side. Flip and cook for another 2 minutes. Add the lemon juice.
5. In a separate small saucepan, combine the spinach and the remaining ¼ cup of water. Steam for about 2 minutes, until the spinach is wilted.
6. Remove the sweet potato skin and mash the sweet potato with a fork. Divide the sweet potato between two bowls, then add the quinoa, spinach, and chickpeas. Spread the pickled onions over the top. Drizzle with the tahini dressing and garnish the scallops with a wedge of lemon.

COOKING TIP: Because this dish has multiple parts, it's best to have all the ingredients measured out, cleaned or rinsed, and set up before starting.

Per serving: Calories: 656; Fat: 26g; Sodium: 683mg; Carbohydrates: 79g; Fiber: 12g; Sugar: 18g; Protein: 29g

Seaside Fish Stew

Prep time: 10 minutes | Cook time: 15 minutes | Serves: 2

Quick, One Pot, Dairy-Free, Gluten-Free

This stew makes you feel like you should be sitting by the ocean. White fish is a great source of vitamin B_{12} and niacin, not to mention that it is a great source of protein. The cooked tomatoes provide lycopene, which is considered a powerful antioxidant that helps fight certain types of cancer. The stew is great with sautéed spinach or on top of brown rice.

- 2 tablespoons olive oil
- ¾ cup chopped onion
- 1 garlic clove, minced
- ¼ cup chopped green bell pepper
- 2 tablespoons chopped celery
- 2 tablespoons chopped carrot
- ¼ cup white wine
- ½ cup low-sodium chicken broth
- ¾ cup chopped plum tomatoes
- 4 ounces tomato sauce
- 4 ounces cod fillets, cubed
- 4 ounces scallops (halved if they are large)
- 4 ounces halibut fillets, cubed
- ¾ teaspoon Italian seasoning
- ¾ teaspoon salt
- ¼ teaspoon freshly ground black pepper
- Chopped fresh chives, for garnish

1. In a 4-quart pot, heat the oil over medium heat and sauté the onion and garlic until translucent. Add the bell pepper, celery, and carrot, and continue cooking for about 2 minutes, until the vegetables soften.
2. Add the wine and cook until reduced by half. Add the broth and cook for another 2 minutes on medium-low heat.
3. Add the tomatoes and tomato sauce, cook for another 1 minute, and then add the cod, scallops, halibut, Italian seasoning, salt, and pepper.
4. Cook until the fish is flaky, 7 to 8 minutes on low to medium heat. Do not bring to a boil.
5. Serve in bowls and garnish with chopped chives.

SUBSTITUTION TIP: If you do not have this combination of fish, you can use red snapper, sea bass, shrimp, or any firm white fish.

Per serving: Calories: 354; Fat: 15g; Sodium: 1,217mg; Carbohydrates: 18g; Fiber: 3.5g; Sugar: 8g; Protein: 31g

Baked Halibut and Asparagus

Prep time: 10 minutes | Cook time: 10 minutes | Serves: 2

Halibut is a great fish option for clean eating because it has a sturdy meat-like texture. It is lower in calories and fat but still a great source of protein. The asparagus contains vitamins C and A, which are great for the skin as well as to fight off inflammation.

- 2 (6-ounce) pieces halibut, rinsed and patted dry
- 8 ounces asparagus, trimmed
- ½ teaspoon salt
- Freshly ground black pepper
- 1½ teaspoons freshly squeezed lemon juice
- 1 teaspoon olive oil
- ¼ cup plain low-fat Greek yogurt
- ¼ teaspoon grated lemon zest
- ½ teaspoon chopped shallot
- ¼ teaspoon dried thyme
- 2 tablespoons grated Parmesan cheese
- 10 cherry tomatoes, halved
- 2 lemon wedges, garnish

1. Preheat the oven to 425°F. Line a baking sheet with parchment paper.
2. Put the halibut and asparagus on the prepared baking sheet. Season with the salt and pepper to taste. Pour the lemon juice over the halibut and the oil over the asparagus. Bake for 6 minutes or until the fish is firm.
3. In a small bowl, combine the yogurt, lemon zest, shallot, and thyme, and mix well. When the fish is ready, remove the pan from the oven, spread the yogurt mixture on top, and sprinkle with the Parmesan cheese.
4. Place the tomatoes on the baking sheet with the fish and asparagus and broil on high for 2 minutes, until the Parmesan cheese is golden.
5. Serve with the lemon wedges for garnish.

COOKING TIP: Be sure to not overcook the fish or it will dry out. Oven temperatures vary, so you may not need to cook it for the full 6 minutes.

Per serving: Calories: 234; Fat: 6.5g; Sodium: 799mg; Carbohydrates: 8g; Fiber: 2.5g; Sugar: 4.5g; Protein: 35g

Salmon with Coconut Sauce

Prep time: 10 minutes | Cook time: 20 minutes | Serves: 2

The full-bodied coconut sauce in this recipe gives this baked salmon dish a four-star-restaurant feel. Salmon, as well as its skin, contains omega-3 fatty acids, which are great for brain and heart health. The arugula is beneficial for liver and bone health.

- 1¼ teaspoons olive oil
- 2 (7-ounce) salmon fillets, rinsed and patted dry
- ¼ cup chopped shallot
- 3 plum tomatoes, chopped
- ¼ cup jarred roasted red peppers
- 1¼ cups vegetable broth
- ¾ cup full-fat coconut milk
- ½ cup frozen peas
- 2 teaspoons chopped fresh chives
- ¾ teaspoon salt
- ¼ teaspoon freshly ground black pepper
- 2½ cups arugula
- ¼ cup shredded Monterey Jack cheese

1. Preheat the oven to 400°F. Line a baking sheet with parchment paper.
2. In a nonstick skillet or sauté pan, heat the oil over high heat and swirl to coat the pan. Add the salmon fillets, skin-side up. Cook for about 2 minutes.
3. Place the seared salmon on the prepared baking sheet and bake for 12 to 15 minutes or until the salmon flakes easily with a fork. (Cooking time may vary depending on fillet thickness.) Transfer to a plate and set aside.
4. In the same pan, sauté the shallot over medium heat for about 1 minute, until the shallot is softened, then add the tomatoes and red peppers and cook for 1 more minute.
5. Add the vegetable broth, reduce the heat to low, and cook until the liquid is reduced by half.

6. Add the coconut milk, peas, and chives, and stir for 30 seconds; add the salt and pepper. Add the arugula and allow to wilt, then stir in the cheese to combine all the ingredients.
7. Place the vegetable mixture on two plates and top each with the salmon.

COOKING TIP: The salmon skin is edible, but if you want to remove it, you can easily take a spatula and slide it between the skin and the fish when you take it off the baking sheet.

Per serving: Calories: 654; Fat: 40g; Sodium: 1,155mg; Carbohydrates: 20g; Fiber: 5.5g; Sugar: 8.5g; Protein: 55g

Sunday Shrimp and Pasta

Prep time: 5 minutes | Cook time: 15 minutes | Serves: 2

Quick

This simple shrimp and pasta dish is very satisfying, and good for you. Shrimp is low calorie and contains omega-3 fatty acids and vitamin B_{12}. The garlic supports your immune system and helps prevent or manage high blood pressure.

- 6 ounces spaghetti or linguine
- ¾ teaspoon salt, divided
- 2 tablespoons olive oil
- 3 ounces asparagus, cut into ½-inch pieces
- 12 ounces shrimp, cleaned and tail shell removed
- 3 garlic cloves, peeled and cut in thirds
- ¼ cup chopped fresh parsley
- 2 tablespoons white wine
- 1 tablespoon freshly squeezed lemon juice
- 2 plum tomatoes, chopped (about 1¼ cups)
- 1½ tablespoons Spinach and Basil Pesto (page 114)
- 1 teaspoon grated Parmesan cheese, for garnish (optional)
- ⅛ teaspoon freshly ground black pepper

1. Fill a 4-quart pot with water and bring to a boil. Add the pasta and ½ teaspoon of salt and cook for 8 to 10 minutes or until al dente.
2. In a nonstick skillet or sauté pan, heat the oil over medium heat. Add the asparagus and cook for 1 minute, then add the shrimp. When the shrimp turns pink on one side, turn them over, add the garlic, and cook for another 30 seconds. Add the parsley and stir. Add the white wine and lemon juice and cook for another 30 seconds. Add the tomatoes and pesto and stir to combine.
3. Divide the pasta into two bowls and top each with half the shrimp mixture. Sprinkle the Parmesan cheese (if using) on top. Season with the remaining ¼ teaspoon of salt and the pepper.

COOKING TIP: Be careful not to overcook the shrimp, as the texture will turn rubbery.

Per serving: Calories: 669; Fat: 23g; Sodium: 1,123mg; Carbohydrates: 71g; Fiber: 4.5g; Sugar: 5g; Protein: 43g

Smoky Baja Fish Tacos

Prep time: 15 minutes | Cook time: 10 minutes | Makes: 6 tacos

A smoky, dairy-free crema sauce and crunchy, tangy slaw elevate these quick and easy Baja fish tacos. This dish will surely become a staple in your weeknight dinner rotation.

- ½ cup unsalted raw cashews
- ½ cup water
- 2 teaspoons freshly squeezed lime juice, divided
- ½ teaspoon smoked paprika
- ½ teaspoon salt, divided
- 1 cup thinly sliced red cabbage
- ¼ cup shredded carrot
- 2 tablespoons thinly sliced red onion
- 2 tablespoons chopped fresh cilantro
- ¼ teaspoon ground cumin
- ⅛ teaspoon chili powder
- ⅛ teaspoon garlic powder
- 10 ounces white fish fillets (cod, halibut, etc.)
- 1 tablespoon olive oil
- 6 corn tortillas

1. In a blender or food processor, combine the cashews, water, 1 teaspoon of lime juice, paprika, and ¼ teaspoon of salt. Blend until smooth and set aside.
2. In a small bowl, combine the cabbage, carrot, onion, cilantro, remaining 1 teaspoon of lime juice, and a pinch of salt, and mix thoroughly. Set aside.
3. In a separate small bowl, combine the cumin, chili powder, garlic powder, and the remaining ¼ teaspoon of salt and mix. Sprinkle the mixture evenly on the fish and gently rub it in.
4. In a medium skillet or sauté pan, heat the oil over medium heat. Once hot, add the fish and cook for 2 to 3 minutes on each side or until it begins to flake.
5. Warm the tortillas in a small skillet or wrap in a damp paper towel and microwave them for 30 seconds.
6. Put three tortillas on each plate and divide the fish evenly between the tortillas. Top with the slaw and smoky crema.

VARIATION TIP: Try making an avocado crema by mashing 1 avocado with ¼ cup of water, 1 tablespoon of lime juice, ½ teaspoon of smoked paprika, and ½ teaspoon of salt.

Per serving (3 tacos): Calories: 443; Fat: 21g; Sodium: 675mg; Carbohydrates: 33g; Fiber: 3.5g; Sugar: 4g; Protein: 31g

Mediterranean Cod with Tapenade

Prep time: 10 minutes | Cook time: 20 minutes | Serves: 2

Quick, Dairy-Free, Gluten-Free

This is a light and airy dish popping with both color and flavor. This dish is on the table quickly and is loaded with nutrients to help fight inflammation and chronic disease. You can serve it with rice or a salad.

- 2 (6-ounce) cod fillets, rinsed and patted dry
- 2 tablespoons olive oil, divided, plus 1 teaspoon
- 8 ounces asparagus, trimmed
- ½ cup chopped kalamata olives
- ½ cup cherry tomatoes, halved
- 1 avocado, cubed (same size as the tomatoes and olives)
- 1 teaspoon capers, drained and rinsed
- 1 tablespoon chopped scallion, white part only
- ½ tablespoon freshly squeezed lemon juice
- ½ teaspoon salt
- ¼ teaspoon freshly ground black pepper
- 1 tablespoon chopped fresh parsley
- 2 lemon wedges, for garnish

1. Preheat the oven to 400°F. Line half a baking sheet with parchment paper.
2. Place the cod on the parchment paper and drizzle with 1 tablespoon of olive oil. Place the asparagus on the other side of the baking sheet and drizzle with 1 teaspoon of olive oil. Season with salt and pepper.
3. Bake for about 20 minutes or until the fish is flaky.
4. In a small bowl, combine the olives, tomatoes, avocado, capers, and scallion. Add the remaining 1 tablespoon of olive oil, the lemon juice, salt, and pepper.
5. Divide the fish and asparagus between two plates and pour the olive mixture over the fish. Sprinkle with the parsley and garnish with the lemon wedges.

VARIATION TIP: Halibut, red snapper, or flounder would work instead of the cod.

Per serving: Calories: 461; Fat: 32g; Sodium: 1,262mg; Carbohydrates: 15g; Fiber: 7.5g; Sugar: 3.5g; Protein: 31g

Squash-Stuffed Sole Fillets

Prep time: 10 minutes | Cook time: 15 minutes | Serves: 2

This stuffed fish is my version of vegetarian sushi, only in this case the wrap is the fish, not the rice! It is low calorie and very tasty. The Parmesan cheese and paprika topping on the rolled fish give it a nice finishing touch.

- 4 ounces zucchini, cut into matchsticks (about 1¼ cups)
- 2 ounces yellow squash, cut into very thin strips (about ½ cup)
- 1 tablespoon freshly squeezed lemon juice
- ½ teaspoon dried thyme
- ¼ teaspoon salt
- ⅛ teaspoon freshly ground black pepper
- 2 (7-ounce) sole fillets, rinsed and patted dry
- 2 teaspoons grated Parmesan cheese
- 1 teaspoon olive oil
- ½ teaspoon paprika, or enough to sprinkle on top of the fish

1. Preheat the oven to 375°F. Line a 6-by-6-inch baking dish with parchment paper.
2. Put the zucchini and squash in a medium bowl. Add the lemon juice, thyme, salt, and pepper.
3. Place the fish fillets on a flat surface and place half the vegetable mixture in the center of each fillet. Take the narrowest end of the fillet and tightly roll it. A toothpick will help hold it together.
4. Carefully transfer the rolled fillets to the prepared baking dish.
5. In a separate small bowl, mix the Parmesan cheese with the olive oil and spread it over the rolled fish. Sprinkle the paprika on top.
6. Put the pan in the oven and bake for 10 to 12 minutes or until the fish is flaky.
7. Serve warm.

COOKING TIP: Slice up the leftover zucchini and squash and sauté in a saucepan with some olive oil, salt, and pepper. Serve the zucchini and squash and a side of rice with this dish.

Per serving: Calories: 161; Fat: 6g; Sodium: 823mg; Carbohydrates: 3g; Fiber: 1g; Sugar: 2g; Protein: 22g

Pistachio-Crusted Scrod with String Beans

Prep time: 5 minutes | Cook time: 15 minutes | Serves: 2

This light but flavorful dish gains a little more fat and a burst of flavor from the pistachios. Pistachios are cholesterol-free and have a substantial amount of vitamin B_6 and potassium. String beans are a low-calorie pairing and the perfect match to go with the flavor of the pistachios.

- 12 ounces scrod fillets, rinsed and patted dry
- 3 teaspoons olive oil, divided
- ½ cup pistachios, chopped
- 1½ tablespoons freshly squeezed lemon juice
- 1 teaspoon butter
- 6 thin lemon peel slices
- 10 ounces string beans, trimmed
- ¼ cup sliced almonds

1. Preheat the oven to 350°F. Line a baking sheet with parchment paper and add the scrod.
2. In a small skillet or sauté pan, heat 2 teaspoons of oil over medium heat and toast the pistachios for 45 seconds. Be sure not to overcook. Add the lemon juice and butter and stir to cook for another 30 seconds, until the nuts are coated and moistened.
3. Top each fillet with half the nut mixture, then with the lemon peel slices. Bake the fish for 8 to 10 minutes or until the fish is flaky and turns white.
4. In a nonstick pan, heat the remaining 1 teaspoon of oil. Add the string beans and sauté for 2 minutes. Add the almonds and toss. Once the almonds are lightly toasted, toss once more and serve.

COOKING TIP: If needed, add a splash of water to the string beans to help cook them a little more.

SUBSTITUTION TIP: You can substitute sole, flounder, or another type of white flaky fish for the scrod.

Per serving: Calories: 483; Fat: 29g; Sodium: 530mg; Carbohydrates: 22g; Fiber: 8.5g; Sugar: 8g; Protein: 37g

Swordfish with Boiled Fingerling Potatoes

Prep time: 10 minutes | Cook time: 20 minutes | Serves: 2

Quick, Dairy-Free, Gluten-Free

Swordfish is considered a meatier fish and helps meet protein requirements. Selenium, a mineral found in swordfish, builds up thyroid, immune, and heart health. Oh, and swordfish is a natural source of vitamin D and has omega-3s, too.

- 6 ounces fingerling potatoes
- 12 ounces swordfish fillets, rinsed and patted dry
- 1 tablespoon freshly squeezed lemon juice, plus 1 teaspoon
- 1 tablespoon Dijon mustard
- 1 tablespoon olive oil
- 1 teaspoon minced shallot
- 1 teaspoon dried parsley
- ½ teaspoon dried rosemary
- ¼ teaspoon dried thyme

1. Preheat the oven to 400°F. Line a 12-by-10-inch baking pan with parchment paper.
2. Fill a 4-quart pot with water, add the potatoes, and bring to a boil. Cook until tender and soft, about 10 minutes.
3. Put the fish in the prepared baking pan and coat with 1 teaspoon of lemon juice. Bake for 10 to 12 minutes or until the fish turns opaque in color and flakes when you poke a fork into it.
4. In a small bowl, mix the mustard, remaining 1 tablespoon of lemon juice, the oil, shallot, parsley, rosemary, and thyme, and stir to combine.
5. Drizzle the mustard mixture on top of the fish. Serve with the potatoes on the side.

SUBSTITUTION TIP: Swap tuna or salmon steak for the swordfish.

Per serving: Calories: 350; Fat: 16g; Sodium: 306mg; Carbohydrates: 16g; Fiber: 2g; Sugar: 1g; Protein: 31g

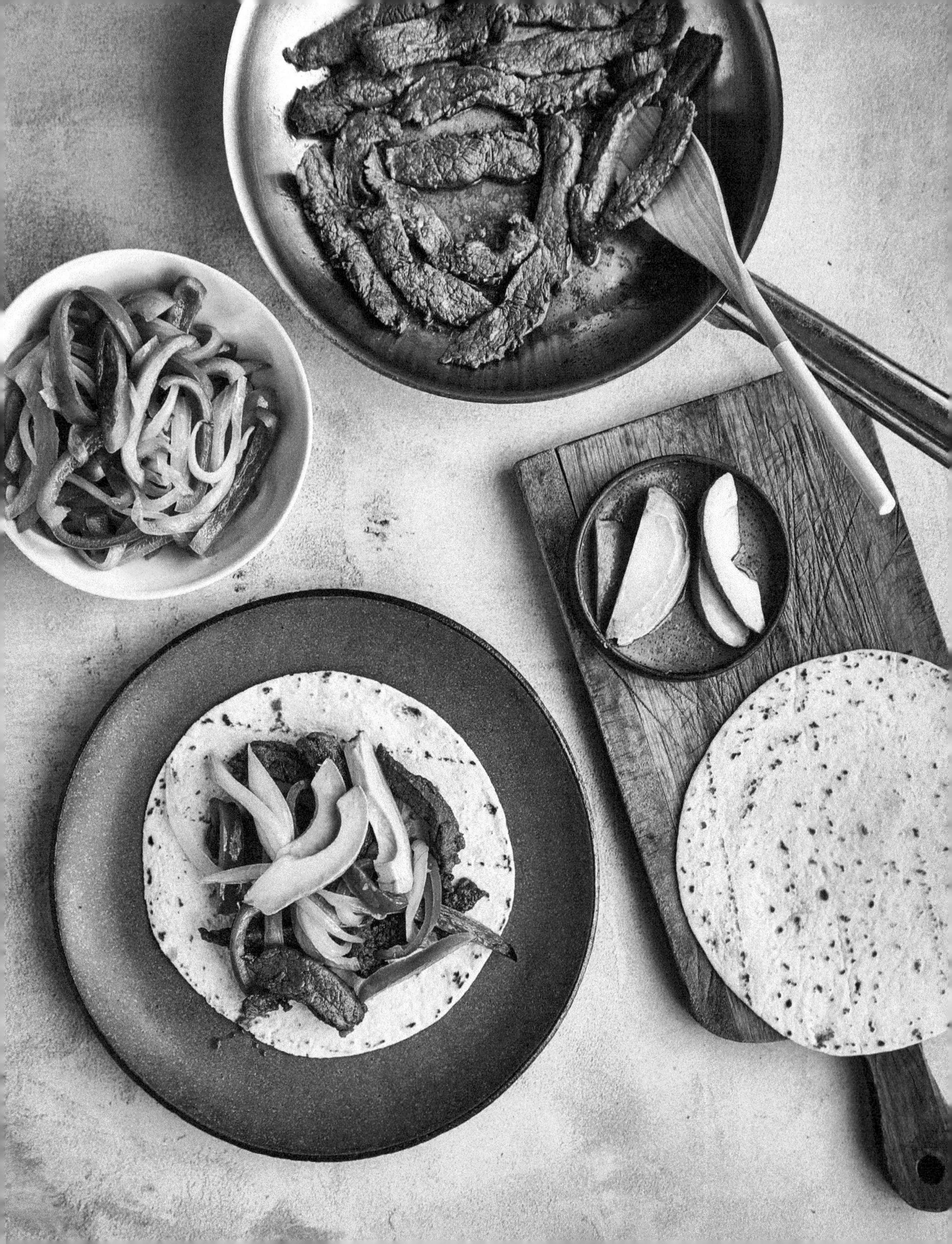

CHAPTER SIX

Poultry and Meat

Speedy Steak Fajitas

Prep time: 10 minutes | Cook time: 10 minutes | Serves: 2

Quick, Dairy-Free, Gluten-Free

Fajitas are a fun way to get in some good lean protein with complex flavors without the need for all-day cooking. You can add some black or pinto beans or brown rice for a bit more carbs if you'd like. For a little healthy fat, slice an avocado and lay the slices on top of the meat and onions. Serve with a side of Salsa (page 119).

- 2¼ teaspoons chili powder
- 2 teaspoons ground cumin
- 2 teaspoons freshly squeezed lemon juice
- 1 teaspoon paprika
- 1 garlic clove, minced
- ¼ teaspoon honey
- ⅛ teaspoon cayenne pepper
- 10 ounces flank steak, thinly sliced
- 3 teaspoons olive oil, divided
- 1 cup sliced onions
- 1 cup sliced green bell peppers
- 2 (10-inch) corn tortillas
- 1 avocado, sliced

1. In a medium bowl, combine the chili powder, cumin, lemon juice, paprika, garlic, honey, and cayenne pepper, and whisk until well combined. Add the flank steak, coat well, and let it marinate while you prepare the onions and peppers.
2. In a skillet or sauté pan, heat 2 teaspoons of oil over medium heat and sauté the onions for 1 minute, until translucent.
3. Add the peppers and cook on medium-high heat for 2 minutes or until soft. Once cooked, transfer the onions and peppers to a small plate.
4. In the same pan, heat the remaining 1 teaspoon of oil over medium-high heat, add the meat, and cook for 4 to 5 minutes or until it is no longer pink.
5. Put the tortillas on a microwaveable plate, cover with a wet paper towel, place in the microwave, and cook for 30 seconds.
6. In the middle of each tortilla, place a portion of the steak and vegetables. Add avocado.
7. Fold each tortilla like a burrito, folding the two sides over the filling and then lifting the bottom flap of the tortilla on top and rolling to fully encase.

Per serving: Calories: 491; Fat: 28g; Sodium: 101mg; Carbohydrates: 28g; Fiber: 8.5g; Sugar: 5.5g; Protein: 33g

Pesto Chicken Thighs with Beans

Prep time: 10 minutes | Cook time: 15 minutes | Serves: 2

The chicken thighs in this recipe offer more flavor than chicken breast while still being a clean and lean protein source. This one-pot meal is a great weekday dish but can also be a wonderful meal to double and serve to guests.

- 1 tablespoon olive oil
- 4 (4-ounce) boneless, skinless chicken thighs
- ½ cup chopped shallots
- 1 cup canned small white beans, rinsed and drained
- 1 plum tomato, chopped
- ⅓ cup oil-packed sun-dried tomatoes, cut into strips
- ¼ cup Spinach and Basil Pesto (page 114)
- ½ teaspoon salt
- ¼ teaspoon freshly ground black pepper

1. In a nonstick skillet or sauté pan, heat the oil over medium heat and swirl to coat the pan. Add the chicken and cook for about 4 minutes. Once brown, turn over and continue cooking for 3 minutes or until cooked through.
2. Reduce the heat to medium, add the shallots, and cook for about 2 minutes, until softened. Add the beans and cook to heat them through, about 1 minute. Add the tomato and cook for 1 minute more.
3. Add the sun-dried tomatoes, cook for another 1 minute, then add the pesto. Season with the salt and pepper.

COOKING TIP: You can substitute chicken breasts for the thighs, but do not use the thin-cut breasts, as they tend to dry out quickly. Cutting the breasts into cubes will decrease the cooking time.

Per serving: Calories: 720; Fat: 37g; Sodium: 1,435mg; Carbohydrates: 40g; Fiber: 9.5g; Sugar: 4.5g; Protein: 59g

One-Skillet Chicken with Olives

Prep time: 10 minutes | Cook time: 15 minutes | Serves: 2

Quick, Dairy-Free

Kalamata olives give this dish a natural saltiness, while the mushrooms give it an umami flavor. The protein found in the chicken is lean, a great choice for clean eating, especially if you have cholesterol issues. I suggest serving it with fingerling potatoes, but rice would work, too.

- 2 tablespoons all-purpose flour
- 12 ounces boneless, skinless chicken breast, cut into 1-inch pieces
- 1½ tablespoons olive oil
- 1 cup sliced mushrooms
- 1 garlic clove, crushed
- 1 teaspoon dried rosemary
- ⅓ cup white wine
- ½ cup low-sodium chicken broth
- ½ cup pitted kalamata olives
- 12 cherry tomatoes
- ¼ teaspoon salt
- ¼ teaspoon freshly ground black pepper
- 1 teaspoon chopped fresh parsley, for garnish

1. Put the flour on a small plate and dredge the chicken pieces in it.
2. In a large nonstick skillet or sauté pan, heat the oil over medium heat. Add the chicken and cook for 5 to 7 minutes, constantly turning to brown on all sides.
3. Add the mushrooms and sauté for about 1 minute, until they begin to soften. Add the garlic and rosemary and continue to cook for about 30 seconds. Pour in the wine and let simmer for 1 minute, then add the broth and cook for another 30 seconds.
4. Add the olives and cherry tomatoes, reduce the heat to low, and simmer for another 1 minute. Season with the salt and pepper and garnish with the parsley.

SUBSTITUTION TIP: Black or green olives can be swapped for the kalamata olives, but doing so will change the taste of the dish slightly.

Per serving: Calories: 490; Fat: 25g; Sodium: 1,076mg; Carbohydrates: 15g; Fiber: 2g; Sugar: 3.5g; Protein: 43g

Turkey and Butter Bean Chili

Prep time: 5 minutes | Cook time: 25 minutes | Serves: 2

Quick, One Pot, Dairy-Free, Gluten-Free

This is a mildly spiced chili that is both flavorful and low in fat and calories. The turkey meat is lean and a good source of protein. Make it ahead of time and use it another day; it keeps in the freezer for up to three months. Serve over rice and top with grated cheese, sliced scallions, and sour cream.

- 1 teaspoon avocado oil
- ½ cup chopped onion
- 8 ounces ground turkey
- 1 garlic clove, minced
- 1 cup canned butter beans, drained and rinsed
- 1 cup canned diced tomatoes with juice
- ⅔ cup tomato sauce
- ½ cup water
- 2 tablespoons chopped jalapeño pepper
- 2 tablespoons chili powder
- 1 tablespoon tomato paste
- 1 teaspoon ground cumin
- 1 bay leaf
- ¼ teaspoon salt
- ¼ teaspoon freshly ground black pepper
- ⅛ teaspoon ground allspice
- Red pepper flakes (optional)

1. In a 4-quart pot, heat the oil over medium heat. Add the onion and sauté for 30 seconds. Add the turkey and garlic and cook for about 5 minutes, until the meat starts to change color and is cooked through.
2. Add the beans, diced tomatoes, tomato sauce, water, jalapeño pepper, chili powder, tomato paste, cumin, bay leaf, salt, pepper, allspice, and red pepper flakes (if using). Stir to combine.
3. Cover with a lid and lower the heat to simmer for another 20 minutes. Remove the bay leaf and discard before serving.

SUBSTITUTION TIP: Substitute ground beef or pork for the turkey if that is what you have on hand.

Per serving: Calories: 382; Fat: 12g; Sodium: 1,404mg; Carbohydrates: 38g; Fiber: 11g; Sugar: 12g; Protein: 31g

Italian Chicken Meatballs

Prep time: 10 minutes | Cook time: 20 minutes | Serves: 2

The small amount of chicken thigh added to the ground chicken in these meatballs adds moisture but still keeps the fat content lower than typical pork or beef meatballs. You can serve these with pasta and marinara sauce or use them as an appetizer. If you want a quick soup, heat some chicken broth, add spinach, and then add the meatballs for additional protein.

- 10 ounces ground chicken
- 2 ounces boneless, skinless chicken thighs, minced
- ¾ cup Italian-seasoned bread crumbs
- ¼ cup grated Parmesan cheese
- 1 large egg
- 2 tablespoons reduced-fat milk
- 1 teaspoon dried parsley
- ¼ teaspoon salt
- Freshly ground black pepper

1. Preheat the oven to 350°F. Line a small baking sheet with parchment paper.
2. In a medium bowl, combine the ground chicken, minced chicken thighs, bread crumbs, Parmesan cheese, egg, milk, parsley, and salt. Season with pepper.
3. Shape the meatballs using about 2 tablespoons of the mixture for each, place the meatballs on the prepared baking sheet, and cook for 10 minutes. Turn the meatballs over and cook for about another 10 minutes, until cooked through.

VARIATION TIP: Make the meatballs smaller—about 1 tablespoon—and serve as an appetizer with Carrot and Cucumber Yogurt Sauce (page 121).

Per serving: Calories: 486; Fat: 20g; Sodium: 1,229mg; Carbohydrates: 31g; Fiber: 3g; Sugar: 4g; Protein: 42g

Shepherd's Pie

Prep time: 10 minutes | Cook time: 25 minutes | Serves: 2

Quick

Growing up with an Irish mother, we always had the traditional lamb in shepherd's pie, but I substituted beef in this recipe. This all-in-one dish is even great to make ahead and have later in the day, or freeze. Serve with a side salad.

- 12 ounces potatoes, peeled and diced
- ½ teaspoon salt
- 10 ounces lean ground beef (90 percent lean)
- ¾ cup chopped onions
- ¼ cup diced celery
- 1 tablespoon tomato paste
- 1½ cups beef broth
- ½ cup frozen peas
- ½ cup frozen carrots
- 1 teaspoon Worcestershire sauce
- 1½ tablespoons butter, plus 1 teaspoon
- 1 teaspoon all-purpose flour
- 2 tablespoons reduced-fat or whole milk
- ¾ teaspoon salt
- ½ teaspoon freshly ground black pepper

1. Preheat the broiler on high.
2. Put the potatoes and salt in a 2-quart pot, cover them with water, and bring to a boil. Reduce the heat to medium and cook until the potatoes are tender, about 10 minutes. Drain and set aside.
3. In a 4-quart pot, sauté the beef on medium heat for 5 to 7 minutes. Once it's browned, drain the fat and transfer the beef to a plate.
4. In the same pot the beef was cooked in, sauté the onions and celery over medium heat for about 2 minutes, until soft. Add the cooked meat back to the pot and cook for 30 seconds. Add the tomato paste and stir. Add the broth, peas, carrots, and Worcestershire sauce, and cook for 1 minute more.
5. In a small microwaveable bowl, melt 1 teaspoon of butter on low for 30 seconds. Add the flour and mix, making a roux. Add the roux to the meat mixture. Combine and cook for another 2 minutes.

CONTINUED

6. Add the milk and remaining 1½ tablespoons of butter to the pot the potatoes were cooked in, allowing the butter to melt. Add the potatoes back to the pot and mash, then add the salt and pepper.
7. Place the meat in an oven-safe dish and gently scoop the mashed potatoes on top. Place under the broiler on high and cook for 1 to 2 minutes until the potatoes start to brown. Serve hot.

SUBSTITUTION TIP: Go the traditional style and use lamb. Ground turkey or chicken would work too, but you'd want to use chicken broth instead of beef broth.

Per serving: Calories: 567; Fat: 25g; Sodium: 1,528mg; Carbohydrates: 46g; Fiber: 9g; Sugar: 11g; Protein: 37g

Pork and Eggplant Marsala

Prep time: 10 minutes | Cook time: 20 minutes | Serves: 2

This lean pork dish is paired with eggplant, which is high in fiber and low in calories and carbs. Try serving with a side of baby red potatoes, or swap the potatoes for another vegetable, or serve it with a simple salad.

12 ounces pork loin, trimmed and flattened
½ cup all-purpose flour
Salt
Freshly ground black pepper
2½ tablespoons olive oil, divided
6 ounces eggplant, chopped
½ cup chopped shallots
4 ounces white mushrooms, sliced
½ cup marsala wine, divided
1 tablespoon freshly squeezed lemon juice
1 teaspoon canned light coconut milk
1 tablespoon water
1 tablespoon chopped fresh rosemary

1. Trim the white ligaments from the pork loin and cut into ½-inch-thick slices. Flatten each slice with a meat tenderizer or rolling pin into a thin fillet.
2. Place the flour on a large plate, season with salt and pepper, and dredge each pork piece in flour, coating both sides.
3. In a nonstick skillet or sauté pan, heat 1½ tablespoons of oil over medium heat and swirl to coat. Add the eggplant and shallots and sauté on medium-high heat for about 1 minute, then add the mushrooms. Once the mushrooms begin to soften after 4 or 5 minutes, transfer the vegetables to a small bowl and set aside.
4. Add the remaining 1 tablespoon of oil to the pan, add the pork, and cook on one side until brown, 4 to 5 minutes. Turn the meat over and cook for 2 minutes, then add the vegetable mixture.
5. Pour ¼ cup of marsala wine and the lemon juice into the pan. Cook for 30 seconds.
6. Add the coconut milk and stir. Add the water, the remaining ¼ cup of marsala wine, and the rosemary. Cook for 30 seconds more, until the pork is cooked through, and serve warm.

USE IT UP: You can grill leftover pork with teriyaki sauce to top a salad or a sandwich.

Per serving: Calories: 680; Fat: 36g; Sodium: 431mg; Carbohydrates: 35g; Fiber: 4.5g; Sugar: 11g; Protein: 42g

Lamb and Vegetable Kabobs

Prep time: 10 minutes | Cook time: 15 minutes | Serves: 2

Quick, Dairy-Free, Gluten-Free

Kabobs are a classic summer grilling dish, but they're perfect for all seasons when roasted in your oven. Feel free to swap out the bell pepper, onion, and tomatoes for other favorite combinations like zucchini and eggplant or serve them wrapped in a flat bread. Serve with the Carrot and Cucumber Yogurt Sauce (page 121) but note that has dairy.

- ½ tablespoon olive oil, plus ¾ teaspoon
- ½ tablespoon freshly squeezed lemon juice
- 1 tablespoon ground cumin, divided
- 1 teaspoon Dijon mustard
- 1 garlic clove, minced
- Pinch salt
- Pinch freshly ground black pepper
- 12 ounces lamb loin, cubed
- ½ tablespoon paprika
- ½ red bell pepper, cut into 1-inch square pieces
- ¼ medium onion, cut into 1-inch slices
- 12 to 15 cherry tomatoes
- 1 tablespoon chopped fresh mint

1. Preheat the oven to 400°F. If using wooden skewers, soak them in water for 30 minutes.
2. In a medium bowl, combine ½ tablespoon of oil, the lemon juice, ½ tablespoon of cumin, the mustard, garlic, salt, and pepper, and whisk to combine. Add the lamb and mix thoroughly. Marinate for 5 minutes or until the oven is heated. Thread the lamb onto four skewers, leaving a little space between each piece on the skewers, and set on a baking sheet and place in the oven. Cook for about 15 minutes, turning them halfway through.
3. In a small skillet or sauté pan, combine the remaining ½ tablespoon of cumin and the paprika and toast on medium heat for 30 seconds, until fragrant. Add the remaining ¾ teaspoon of oil, the bell pepper, and onion. Season with salt and pepper. Sauté for about 1 minute or until the peppers are beginning to soften. Add the cherry tomatoes and stir in the mint.
4. Place the vegetables on a plate and top with the skewers. Serve warm.

COOKING TIP: The length of cooking time may vary depending on the thickness of the lamb cubes. When turning the skewers over halfway through, check for doneness.

Per serving: Calories: 464; Fat: 33g; Sodium: 297mg; Carbohydrates: 9g; Fiber: 2.5g; Sugar: 5g; Protein: 32g

Stovetop Chicken with Sweet Potatoes

Prep time: 10 minutes | Cook time: 15 minutes | Serves: 2

The shiitake mushrooms in this chicken dish add umami flavor and are considered anti-inflammatory, while the coconut milk adds a natural sweetness that helps marry all the flavors together. This is one of my family's favorite dishes.

- 1 tablespoon avocado oil
- 12 ounces boneless, skinless chicken thighs
- ½ cup sliced shiitake mushrooms
- ¼ cup low-sodium chicken broth
- ¼ cup white wine
- 1 tablespoon all-purpose flour
- 1 sweet potato
- ¼ cup canned light coconut milk
- ½ teaspoon salt
- ¼ teaspoon freshly ground black pepper
- 1 tablespoon dried or chopped fresh parsley

1. In a nonstick skillet or sauté pan, heat the oil over medium-high heat. Add the chicken and cook for about 3 minutes to brown on one side. Turn the chicken over and cook for another 2 to 3 minutes.
2. Lower the heat to medium, add the mushrooms, and cook for 1 to 2 minutes.
3. In a small bowl, combine the broth and wine and carefully whisk in the flour. Add the mixture to the pan with the chicken. Cook for 1 minute or until the sauce reduces and thickens slightly.
4. Cook the sweet potato in the microwave for 4 to 5 minutes on high heat. It will be cooked when it's soft on the inside when poked with a fork.
5. To the pan with the chicken, stir in the coconut milk and simmer for another 1 to 2 minutes. Season with the salt and pepper. Use the parsley as garnish. Divide the chicken and sweet potato between two plates and serve.

COOKING TIP: If using dried parsley, add it with the mushrooms; if using fresh parsley add it at the end as a garnish. Chicken thighs can have a little extra fat on the edges, so be sure to trim it off before cooking.

Per serving: Calories: 380; Fat: 15g; Sodium: 785mg; Carbohydrates: 19g; Fiber: 2.5g; Sugar: 4g; Protein: 37g

Spiced Chicken Strips

Prep time: 10 minutes | Cook time: 6 minutes | Serves: 2

Moist and delicious, these chicken strips are a finger food that's still clean eating. They're also an ideal weekday dinner because they're quick to make. Serve with a salad or with a side of roasted carrots, or try with a drizzle of Coconut Dressing with Honey and Lime (page 117).

- ½ teaspoon paprika
- ½ teaspoon garlic powder
- ½ teaspoon onion powder
- 12 ounces chicken breast tenderloins
- 1 tablespoon avocado oil, plus 1 teaspoon (if needed)
- ¼ teaspoon dried oregano
- ¼ teaspoon dried basil
- ⅛ teaspoon salt
- ⅛ teaspoon freshly ground black pepper
- 3 tablespoons freshly squeezed lemon juice

1. In a small bowl, combine the paprika, garlic powder, and onion powder.
2. Lay the chicken strips on a plate and sprinkle the spice mixture over them. Turn over and sprinkle the other side.
3. In a nonstick skillet or sauté pan, heat 1 tablespoon of avocado oil over medium-high heat, swirling to coat. Add the chicken and cook until browned, about 2 minutes. Turn the chicken over and cook for another 2 minutes, until browned. (You may need to add the remaining 1 teaspoon of oil if the pan is too dry.) Add the oregano, basil, salt, and pepper.
4. Add the lemon juice and cook for about 2 minutes or until the liquid has evaporated and the chicken has an internal temperature of 165°F or is no longer pink.

SUBSTITUTION TIP: Try using ground turmeric instead of the paprika, or add fresh garlic instead of the garlic powder.

Per serving: Calories: 249; Fat: 11g; Sodium: 227mg; Carbohydrates: 1g; Fiber: 0g; Sugar: 0.5g; Protein: 34g

Sausage and Broccolini Flatbreads

Prep time: 10 minutes | Cook time: 10 minutes | Serves: 2

This is an all-in-one flatbread dish that is quick, tasty, and nutrient dense, with a mix of protein, carbs, and vegetables to keep you feeling full. Broccolini contains vitamins A and C, both of which ward off the effects of aging and fight inflammation.

- 12 ounces fresh chicken or turkey sausage, removed from casing
- 1½ tablespoons olive oil
- 4 ounces broccolini, chopped
- 2 (7-inch) round flatbreads
- 3 tablespoons Spinach and Basil Pesto (page 114)
- ¾ cup shredded low-moisture part-skim mozzarella cheese

1. Preheat the oven to 350°F.
2. In a nonstick skillet or sauté pan, sauté the sausage over medium heat, breaking it up with a wooden spoon, for 4 to 5 minutes.
3. In a separate small nonstick pan, heat the oil and sauté the broccolini for about 1 minute, until it begins to wilt but does not lose its bright green color.
4. To assemble, place the flatbreads on a baking sheet and spread the pesto on each piece (about 1½ tablespoons for each piece). Top with the sausage and broccolini. Sprinkle the mozzarella over the entire flatbread.
5. Put the flatbreads in the oven and cook for 3 to 4 minutes or until the cheese melts.

COOKING TIP: You can make these ahead of time and store them fully baked in the refrigerator for up to 3 days.

Per serving: Calories: 798; Fat: 46g; Sodium: 1,757mg; Carbohydrates: 46g; Fiber: 6g; Sugar: 4g; Protein: 49g

Turkey-Stuffed Bell Peppers

Prep time: 15 minutes | Cook time: 30 minutes | Serves: 2

These low-carb peppers have a chili-like flavor from the spices used for the turkey. A lean protein dish that is an easy midweek meal, these are also great for lunch the next day. Serve half of each color of bell pepper along with the Kale and Apple Salad (page 40).

1 yellow bell pepper
1 orange bell pepper
1 teaspoon olive or avocado oil
½ cup chopped onions
1 garlic clove, minced
12 ounces ground turkey
1 teaspoon chili powder
½ teaspoon ground cumin
¼ teaspoon paprika
⅛ teaspoon salt
Freshly ground black pepper
1¼ cups tomato sauce, divided
½ cup shredded Cheddar cheese
2 scallions, white parts only, for garnish

1. Preheat the oven to 400°F.
2. Cut the peppers in half lengthwise, clean out the seeds, and remove the stems. Place on a baking sheet and cook for 5 to 8 minutes, until the peppers are slightly soft. When done, set aside.
3. In a nonstick pan, heat the oil over medium-high heat. Add the onions and garlic and sauté for 1 minute, until the onions begin to soften. Add the turkey and cook for another 30 seconds.
4. Add the chili powder, cumin, paprika, salt, pepper to taste, and ½ cup of tomato sauce, and sauté until the meat is cooked through.
5. Into an 8-by-8-inch baking pan, pour about ½ cup of tomato sauce and spread to cover the bottom of the pan.
6. Carefully stuff each pepper with the meat mixture and top each with the remaining ¼ cup of tomato sauce.
7. Top with the cheese and put back in the oven for 20 minutes, until the cheese is melted and lightly browned. Garnish with the scallions and serve.

COOKING TIP: Have the turkey meat crumbled before cooking. The small crumbles fit better in the peppers.

Per serving: Calories: 506; Fat: 25g; Sodium: 1,283mg; Carbohydrates: 28g; Fiber: 4.5g; Sugar: 15g; Protein: 45g

Spicy Thai Chicken Lettuce Cups

Prep time: 10 minutes | Cook time: 15 minutes | Serves: 2

Quick, Dairy-Free, Gluten-Free

This recipe was inspired by the Thai dish beef larb. It calls for a Thai chile, but you can use a milder chile, like a banana or cherry chile pepper, or omit altogether if you prefer.

- 1 tablespoon avocado oil
- 1 shallot, minced
- 1 Thai chile, sliced
- 1 garlic clove, minced
- 1 pound ground chicken breast
- ½ cucumber, diced
- ¼ cup chopped fresh cilantro
- 4 tablespoons freshly squeezed lime juice, divided
- ¼ teaspoon salt
- 2 tablespoons reduced-sodium tamari
- 2 tablespoons water
- 1 tablespoon fish sauce
- 1 tablespoon honey
- 1 Bibb or butter lettuce head, leaves removed

1. In a large skillet or sauté pan, heat the oil over medium heat. Add the shallot, chile, and garlic, and cook for 2 to 3 minutes, until soft.
2. Add the ground chicken, stir, and cook through, about 4 minutes.
3. In a small bowl, combine the cucumber, cilantro, 2 tablespoons of lime juice, and salt, and mix to combine. Set aside.
4. Once the chicken is cooked through, add the tamari, water, fish sauce, and honey, and stir to combine. Add the remaining 2 tablespoons of lime juice. Cook until the liquid has been absorbed and the chicken begins to brown a bit, about 7 minutes.
5. Place four or five lettuce leaves on each plate. Remove the skillet from the heat and spoon the chicken mixture into each leaf. Top with the cucumber mixture and serve.

SUBSTITUTION TIP: You can use soy sauce in place of tamari, but the dish will no longer be gluten-free. You can also make this with ground turkey or beef if preferred.

Per serving: Calories: 391; Fat: 10g; Sodium: 1,855mg; Carbohydrates: 18g; Fiber: 1.5g; Sugar: 12g; Protein: 56g

Apple-Sage Turkey Burgers

Prep time: 10 minutes | Cook time: 25 minutes | Makes: 2 burgers

These turkey burgers are packed with flavor, and with the help of the apple, they are also quite juicy. A quick and easy honey mustard sauce adds tang and sweetness to this savory and lean burger.

- 8 ounces ground turkey
- ½ apple, grated
- 1 garlic clove, minced
- ½ teaspoon ground sage
- ½ teaspoon dried thyme
- ½ teaspoon salt, plus more for seasoning
- ¼ teaspoon onion powder
- ¼ teaspoon freshly ground black pepper, plus more for seasoning
- 1 large sweet potato, cut into rounds
- 1 teaspoon avocado oil
- 2 teaspoons Dijon mustard
- 2 teaspoons honey

1. Preheat the oven to 350°F. Line a baking sheet with parchment paper.
2. In a large bowl, combine the turkey, apple, garlic, sage, thyme, salt, onion powder, and pepper, and mix to combine well.
3. Divide the mixture in half and shape into two patties, placing them on half the baking sheet. Place the sweet potato rounds on the other half and drizzle with the oil and season with salt and pepper.
4. Bake for 20 to 25 minutes or until the burgers reach an internal temperature of 165°F and the sweet potatoes are tender.
5. In a small bowl, mix the mustard and honey together.
6. Serve each burger with half of the sweet potato and top each burger with half of the honey mustard.

COOKING TIP: If you prefer you can also pan sear the burgers, cooking them until they reach an internal temperature of 165°F.

Per serving (1 burger): Calories: 308; Fat: 11g; Sodium: 811mg; Carbohydrates: 29g; Fiber: 3.5g; Sugar: 13g; Protein: 24g

Thyme-Roasted Pork Tenderloin

Prep time: 5 minutes | Cook time: 30 minutes | Serves: 2

This simple, quick, and tasty pork tenderloin recipe is sure to become a favorite. Pork tenderloin is low in saturated fat, making it an excellent protein to add variety to your diet.

- 1 tablespoon olive oil
- 1 small shallot, finely diced
- 1 teaspoon dried thyme
- ½ teaspoon salt
- ½ teaspoon garlic powder
- ½ teaspoon onion powder
- ½ teaspoon ground coriander
- ½ teaspoon paprika
- ¼ teaspoon freshly ground black pepper
- 1 pound pork tenderloin

1. Preheat the oven to 425°F.
2. In a large skillet or sauté pan, heat the oil over medium heat and cook the shallot for 2 to 3 minutes, until softened.
3. Meanwhile, in a small bowl, mix the thyme, salt, garlic powder, onion powder, coriander, paprika, and pepper. Rub the mixture on the pork tenderloin until it is fully coated.
4. Add the tenderloin to the skillet and sear on all sides, about 2 minutes per side.
5. Transfer the tenderloin to a baking dish and bake for 20 minutes or until it reaches an internal temperature of 145°F.
6. Remove from the oven and let rest for 15 minutes before slicing and serving.

COOKING TIP: While searing the pork tenderloin in the pan, try to coat it with the shallot to create an extra-crispy crust.

Per serving: Calories: 301; Fat: 12g; Sodium: 677mg; Carbohydrates: 0g; Fiber: 0g; Sugar: 0g; Protein: 44g

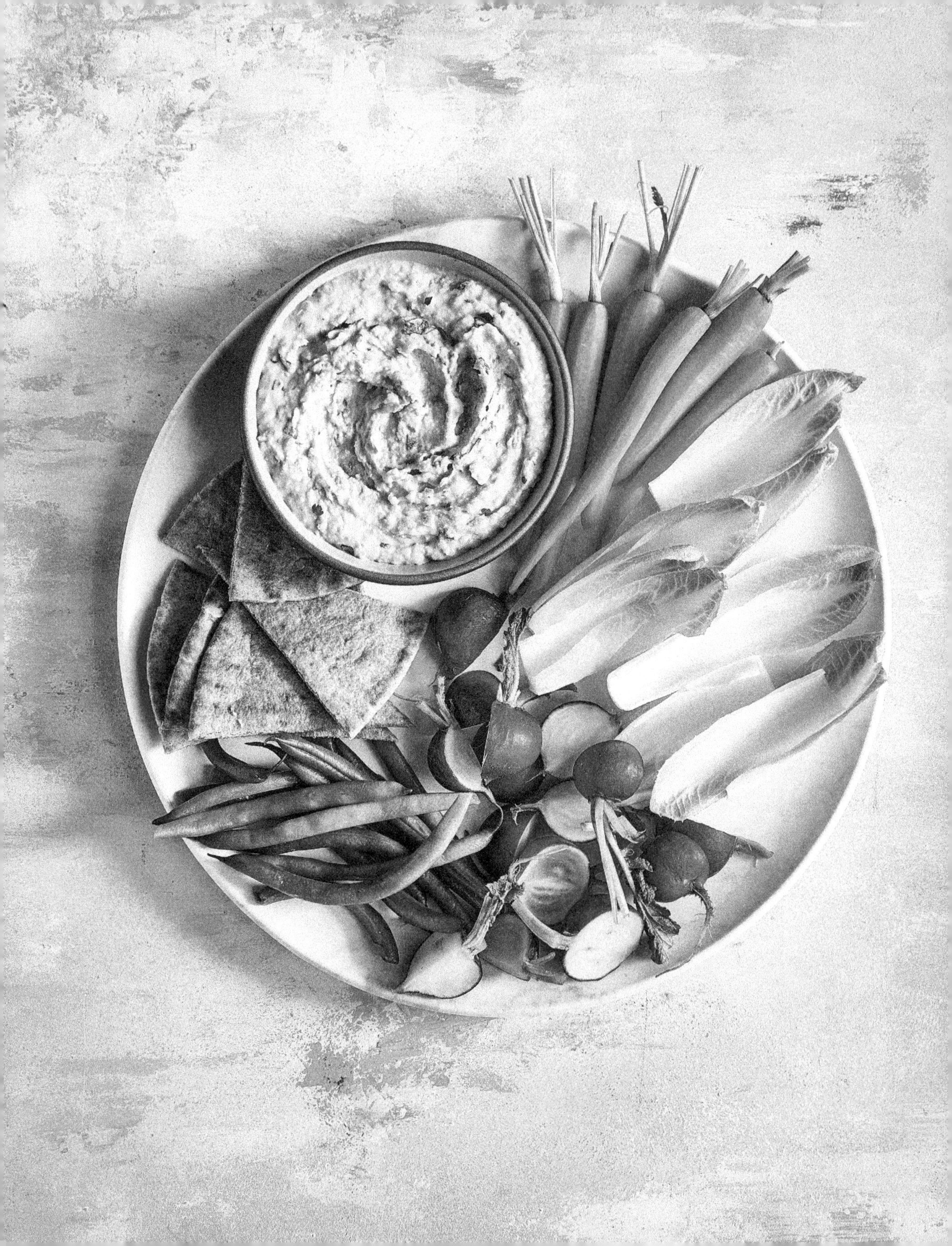

CHAPTER SEVEN

Snacks and Desserts

Roasted and Toasted Seeds and Chickpeas

Prep time: 5 minutes | Cook time: 25 minutes | Makes: 2 cups

Quick, 5-Ingredient, Gluten-Free, Vegan

This snack offers that satisfying crunch we sometimes crave from potato chips. Pumpkin seeds are a healthy fat and provide lots of lean protein, and they also help reduce chronic inflammation. Sesame seeds are immune boosting as well, so this is a win-win snack and a fantastic substitute for a salty or crunchy chip.

- 1 (15-ounce) can chickpeas, drained and rinsed
- 4 tablespoons olive oil
- ¼ cup pumpkin seeds
- ¼ cup sesame seeds
- 2 teaspoons freshly squeezed lemon juice
- ⅛ teaspoon salt

1. Preheat the oven to 425°F. Line a baking sheet with parchment paper.
2. After draining and rinsing the chickpeas, place them on a pan or plate and pat dry with a towel.
3. In a bowl, combine the chickpeas and oil and stir to combine. Place on the prepared baking sheet in a single layer. Cook for 20 to 25 minutes, stirring every 10 minutes, until the color of the chickpeas darkens a little.
4. Meanwhile, in a nonstick skillet or sauté pan, toast the pumpkin and sesame seeds over medium heat for about 1 minute. If the seeds start to pop, take them off the heat.
5. Once the chickpeas are done, take them out and place them in a bowl. Add the toasted seeds and toss with the lemon juice and salt.

COOKING TIP: Be sure to not overcook the chickpeas; they might end up having a bitter taste.

SUBSTITUTION TIP: If you want more spice, try adding paprika and celery salt, or some of your favorite spices.

Per serving (1 cup): Calories: 503; Fat: 37g; Sodium: 396mg; Carbohydrates: 30g; Fiber: 8.5g; Sugar: 5g; Protein: 17g

White Bean and Cilantro Hummus

Prep time: 5 minutes | Makes: 2 cups

Quick, Gluten-Free, Vegan

This is a great snack that can be served with pita bread, celery and carrot slices, or with any of your favorite sliced vegetables. The more colorful the vegetables are, the more the variety of nutrients you are consuming. This is a snack that will keep well in your refrigerator for a few days, so don't feel like you have to eat it all at once.

- 1 garlic clove, peeled
- 1 (15-ounce) can small white beans, drained and rinsed
- 4 tablespoons freshly squeezed lemon juice
- 2 tablespoons olive oil
- 2 tablespoons tahini
- 2 tablespoons cold water
- 2 tablespoons chopped fresh cilantro
- 1 teaspoon maple syrup
- ¾ teaspoon salt
- ¼ teaspoon freshly ground black pepper

1. Put the garlic in the food processor and pulse until minced. Add the beans and pulse again for 30 seconds or until the beans start to puree.
2. Add the lemon juice, oil, tahini, water, cilantro, and maple syrup. Process until the mixture is smooth and well blended. Add the salt and pepper and mix well.

Per serving (¼ cup): Calories: 147; Fat: 6g; Sodium: 221mg; Carbohydrates: 17g; Fiber: 7.5g; Sugar: 1.5g; Protein: 6g

Whipped Avocado Eggs

Prep time: 10 minutes | Cook time: 10 minutes | Serves: 2

This is an alternative to classic deviled eggs, but with lots of bright color and healthy fats. The fresh cilantro brings anti-inflammatory properties, and I love that little crunch from the almond bits. This snack is good for any time of the day.

- 4 large eggs
- 1 avocado, peeled and pitted
- 2 tablespoons chopped fresh cilantro
- 1 teaspoon almonds, finely chopped
- 1 teaspoon freshly squeezed lime juice
- ¼ teaspoon salt
- ¼ teaspoon freshly ground black pepper

1. Fill a small pot with water, enough to cover the eggs with 1 inch of water. Bring the eggs to a boil and continue to boil for about 10 minutes. Once they are cooked, put the eggs into an ice water bath to cool off, then peel.
2. While the eggs are cooking, in a small bowl, mash the avocado. Add the cilantro, almonds, lime juice, salt, and pepper, and mix well.
3. Cut the eggs in half lengthwise and remove the egg yolks.
4. Spoon the avocado mixture into each egg white.

SUBSTITUTION TIP: If you don't like cilantro, use parsley or chives instead.

VARIATION TIP: Try mixing the yolk in with the avocado mixture for an even richer filling.

Per serving: Calories: 265; Fat: 21g; Sodium: 439mg; Carbohydrates: 7g; Fiber: 5g; Sugar: 0.5g; Protein: 14g

Quick, 5-Ingredient, Gluten-Free, Vegetarian

No-Crust Pizza Roll-Ups

Prep time: 10 minutes | Cook time: 10 minutes | Makes: 6 roll-ups

This is a low-carb snack with all the flavor of pizza but without the guilt. Choose a different vegetable for the topping if you have something else in your refrigerator. If you don't finish these in one sitting, keep them in the refrigerator for the next day.

- 1 cup shredded low-moisture part-skim mozzarella cheese
- ¼ cup tomato sauce
- ¼ teaspoon dried oregano
- ¼ cup chopped broccoli florets

1. Preheat the oven to 450°F. Line a baking sheet with parchment paper.
2. Sprinkle the mozzarella cheese onto the parchment paper, dividing the cheese into six small even circles.
3. In a small bowl, combine the tomato sauce and oregano, and stir. Spoon a little tomato sauce on each of the cheese circles and top with the broccoli.
4. Bake for 7 minutes or until the edges of the cheese start to brown.
5. Remove from the oven and let cool for 1 minute or until you can handle them. Roll them up and serve.

Per serving (3 roll-ups): Calories: 180; Fat: 11g; Sodium: 550mg; Carbohydrates: 6g; Fiber: 0.5g; Sugar: 3g; Protein: 14g

Green Bean Fries

Prep time: 10 minutes | Cook time: 15 minutes | Serves: 2

Whether your diet is plant based or not, this is a great snack when you are looking for a little crunch. The dipping sauce gives the fries the finishing touch with a sweet-and-sour combo.

For the beans

5 ounces string beans
1 large egg
⅓ cup all-purpose flour
¼ teaspoon salt, plus more for seasoning
⅛ teaspoon freshly ground black pepper

For the dipping sauce

3 tablespoons coconut aminos
1½ teaspoons rice vinegar
1½ teaspoons honey

To prepare the beans

1. Preheat the oven to 450°F. Line a baking sheet with parchment paper.
2. Wash the string beans, cut off the ends, and pat them dry.
3. In a small bowl, whisk the egg. In a separate bowl, combine the flour, salt, and pepper.
4. Put a few string beans at a time in the flour and shake off the excess flour. Then coat the beans with the egg and put them on the baking sheet. Repeat this step until all the string beans are coated with flour and egg.
5. Bake for 13 minutes or until the batter is turning brown. Season with salt.

To make the dipping sauce

6. In a small bowl, mix the coconut aminos, rice vinegar, and honey. Serve with the baked green beans.

SUBSTITUTION TIP: To make this gluten-free, swap your favorite gluten-free brand for the all-purpose flour, or use rice flour or almond flour.

Per serving: Calories: 124; Fat: 2g; Sodium: 582mg; Carbohydrates: 22g; Fiber: 2g; Sugar: 11g; Protein: 5g

Sweet Potato Cookies with Raisins and Pecans

Prep time: 10 minutes | Cook time: 15 minutes | Makes: 4 cookies

These cookies require no flour or dairy whatsoever, making them naturally gluten-free and vegetarian—the perfect clean-eating dessert. They pair nicely with some afternoon tea or are great as a midmorning snack.

½ ripe banana
1 tablespoon sugar-free peanut butter
1 tablespoon honey
⅛ teaspoon ground cinnamon
Pinch ground allspice
Pinch salt
½ cup peeled and grated sweet potato
1 tablespoon raisins, divided
1 tablespoon pecans, chopped

1. Preheat the oven to 400°F. Line a baking sheet with parchment paper.
2. In a medium bowl, mash the banana well. Add the peanut butter, honey, cinnamon, allspice, and salt, and stir to combine. Add the sweet potato and mix until fully coated. Fold in half the raisins and all the pecans.
3. Scoop four mounds of the mixture onto the baking sheet and press down lightly on each one to form a cookie shape. Add the remaining raisins to the cookies in the centers, pressing down.
4. Bake for 15 minutes or until slightly firm and browned around the edges. Remove from the oven and cool completely before enjoying.

USE IT UP: Have leftover Golden Spiced Granola (page 25)? Try folding it into these cookies in place of the raisins and pecans so it won't go to waste.

Per serving (2 cookies): Calories: 178; Fat: 6.5g; Sodium: 123mg; Carbohydrates: 28g; Fiber: 2.5g; Sugar: 16g; Protein: 3g

No-Bake Oat Squares

Prep time: 10 minutes | Makes: 25 squares

Quick, Dairy-Free, Gluten-Free, Vegetarian

Sometimes you have a craving for something sweet, and these oat squares will do the trick while still keeping with you on track with your clean-eating goals. It's a quick snack that you can make and keep in the refrigerator for up to a week. One square does the trick, but you may feel like two is better. Either way, it's all good!

- 1 cup certified gluten-free rolled oats
- ¼ cup sugar-free peanut butter
- ¼ cup dark chocolate chips
- 3 tablespoons coconut oil, melted
- 2 tablespoons hemp seeds
- 2 dates, pitted
- 1½ tablespoons maple syrup
- 1 teaspoon vanilla extract
- ½ teaspoon ground nutmeg

1. Put the oats in a food processor and pulse to break them down a little, but not to the granular level.
2. Add the peanut butter, chocolate chips, coconut oil, hemp seed, dates, maple syrup, vanilla, and nutmeg. Pulse in the food processor until all the ingredients come together.
3. Transfer the mixture to a 5-by-5-inch baking pan and flatten the mixture. Cut into 25 squares.

SUBSTITUTION TIP: If you need these to be vegan, change the chocolate chips to raw cacao chips.

Per serving (1 square): Calories: 66; Fat: 4.5g; Sodium: 8mg; Carbohydrates: 6g; Fiber: 1g; Sugar: 2.5g; Protein: 1g

Quick, Gluten-Free, Vegetarian

Flourless Oatmeal-Raisin Cookies

Prep time: 10 minutes | Cook time: 15 minutes | Makes: 6 cookies

Making a small batch of cookies couldn't be easier, and these oatmeal-raisin ones are top-notch. The oats are great for heart health, and there's none of the added sugar or preservatives typically found in store-bought cookies. These cookies will satisfy those sweet cravings in a healthy way.

- 1¼ cups certified gluten-free rolled oats, divided
- 1 teaspoon baking soda
- ½ teaspoon baking powder
- 1 large egg
- 2 tablespoons plus 2 teaspoons plain low-fat Greek yogurt
- 2½ tablespoons maple syrup
- 1 tablespoon coconut oil, melted
- ¼ teaspoon vanilla extract
- ½ cup raisins

1. Preheat the oven to 350°F. Line a small baking sheet with parchment paper.
2. Place ½ cup of oats in a food processor and pulse until the oats are ground and have a grainy texture.
3. In a medium bowl, mix the ground oats, remaining ¾ cup of oats, baking soda, and baking powder to combine.
4. In a separate bowl, mix the egg, yogurt, maple syrup, coconut oil, and vanilla.
5. Slowly add the dry oat mixture to the yogurt mixture. Fold in the raisins.
6. Spoon the cookie mixture onto the prepared baking sheet to make six equal-size cookies. Bake for 10 to 12 minutes or until the cookies are firm to the touch.

COOKING TIP: These cookies will be completely cooked but won't look as brown as store-bought ones; be sure not to overcook them.

SUBSTITUTION TIP: If you have a chocolate lover in the house, exchange the raisins for chocolate chips or carob chips.

Per serving (3 cookies): Calories: 454; Fat: 11g; Sodium: 770mg; Carbohydrates: 84g; Fiber: 6.5g; Sugar: 41g; Protein: 9g

Peachy Baked Oats

Prep time: 10 minutes | Cook time: 20 minutes | Serves: 2

Quick, Dairy-Free, Gluten-Free, Vegetarian

This is an easy dessert to whip up quickly and enjoy after dinner. Serve with a dollop of plain yogurt and a drop of vanilla extract.

For the peaches

2 cups fresh or frozen sliced peaches
1 tablespoon almond flour
2½ teaspoons honey
1 teaspoon vanilla extract
¼ teaspoon freshly squeezed lemon juice

For the topping

½ cup gluten-free rolled oats
2 tablespoons coconut oil, melted
2 tablespoons pecans, finely chopped
1 tablespoon almond flour
½ teaspoon ground nutmeg

To prepare the peaches

1. Preheat the oven to 350°F.
2. In a small bowl, combine the peaches, almond flour, honey, vanilla, and lemon juice, and stir to combine.

To make the topping

3. In a separate small bowl, combine the oats, coconut oil, pecans, almond flour, and nutmeg. Mix well.
4. Divide the peach mixture between two 4-inch oven-safe dishes and top the dishes with the oat mixture.
5. Bake for about 18 minutes or until the oats are lightly browned.

COOKING TIP: If you want to use only one dish for baking, it may take another minute or two to cook the fruit.

SUBSTITUTION TIP: You can use other fruits like plums or apricots. If you use apples or pears, the cooking time will increase.

Per serving: Calories: 359; Fat: 23g; Sodium: 0mg; Carbohydrates: 35g; Fiber: 5g; Sugar: 18g; Protein: 5g

Fudgy Brownies with Date Caramel

Prep time: 10 minutes | Cook time: 25 minutes | Makes: 2 brownies

Gluten-Free, Vegetarian

These nutrient-dense brownies are finished off with a luscious date caramel.

- 1 ounce unsweetened baking chocolate
- ¼ cup unsweetened canned pumpkin puree
- 1 tablespoon avocado oil
- 1 tablespoon honey
- ½ teaspoon salt
- ¼ teaspoon vanilla extract
- 3 tablespoons water
- 1 tablespoon ground flaxseed
- 2 tablespoons chickpea flour or similar gluten-free flour
- 1 teaspoon dried cranberries
- 1 teaspoon pecans, chopped
- 1 teaspoon chopped pumpkin seeds
- 2 dates, pitted, soaked

1. Preheat the oven to 350°F. Line two wells of a muffin tin with parchment paper or cupcake liners and set aside.
2. In a microwave-safe bowl, heat the baking chocolate in the microwave in 20-second intervals on high heat until fully melted. Stir in the pumpkin, avocado oil, honey, salt, and vanilla.
3. In a small bowl, combine the water and flaxseed and stir to combine until the mixture begins to thicken a bit, then add it to the chocolate mixture.
4. Stir in the chickpea flour and mix until well combined. Fold in the cranberries, pecans, and pumpkin seeds.
5. Divide the brownie batter between the two lined wells. Bake for 20 to 25 minutes, until a fork inserted comes out clean.
6. While the brownies are baking, put the soaked dates with a bit of the soaking liquid in a food processor or blender and blend until a thick paste forms (it does not need to be completely smooth).
7. After baking, let cool completely and drizzle each with the caramel. For even fudgier brownies, chill them in the refrigerator for 2 hours.

VARIATION TIP: Feel free to mix up the nuts and seeds with others, such as walnuts or sunflower seeds. You can also add raisins or some Golden Spiced Granola (page 25).

Per serving (1 brownie): Calories: 299; Fat: 17g; Sodium: 586mg; Carbohydrates: 30g; Fiber: 6.5g; Sugar: 19g; Protein: 5g

Creamy Banana Mini "Cheesecakes"

Prep time: 15 minutes, plus 20 minutes to freeze | Cook time: 5 minutes
Makes: 2 mini cheesecakes

Gluten-Free, Vegan

You will not miss the dairy in this vegan take on classic cheesecake. Instead of being baked, this version is frozen and best enjoyed with a drizzle of melted chocolate (although it will no longer be vegan).

- 2 dates, pitted
- ¼ cup raw pecans
- ¼ cup raw cashews
- 1 medium banana, frozen
- 1 tablespoon all-natural peanut butter
- ⅛ teaspoon ground cinnamon

1. Soak the dates in boiling water for 2 to 3 minutes.
2. While the dates are soaking, in a small skillet, toast the pecans and cashews over medium-low heat, stirring frequently until the nuts become fragrant and are lightly browned, about 5 minutes.
3. Drain the dates and put them in a food processor with the nuts and blend until the mixture is fully combined and a large ball forms.
4. Line the bottom of two wells of a muffin tin with parchment paper or a cupcake liner. Divide the date-nut mixture between the two wells and press the mixture down to form the crust, creating an even layer.
5. In the food processor, combine the banana, peanut butter, and cinnamon, and blend until smooth, scraping down the sides as needed.
6. Divide the banana mixture between the two crusts and put in the freezer for about 20 minutes, then enjoy.

VARIATION TIP: For the chocolate lovers out there, try melting ½ ounce of dark chocolate and drizzling it over the frozen cheesecakes before serving.

SUBSTITUTION TIP: You can swap your favorite seeds and seed butter, such as pumpkin or sunflower, for the nuts and nut butter.

Per serving (1 mini cheesecake): Calories: 310; Fat: 19g; Sodium: 29mg; Carbohydrates: 30g; Fiber: 4.5g; Sugar: 17g; Protein: 6g

Tahini and Crispy Rice Cereal Bars

Prep time: 5 minutes | Cook time: 1 minute, plus time to chill | Serves: 2

Quick, 5-Ingredient, Dairy-Free, Gluten-Free, Vegetarian

This tahini and rice cereal bar is a fantastic and clean alternative to the classic. The honey naturally brings out the sweetness, so there is no need for added sugar. If you cannot find brown rice crisp cereal, you can use regular rice crisp cereal instead.

---

2 tablespoons honey
2 tablespoons tahini
⅛ teaspoon ground cinnamon
Pinch ground cardamom
Pinch salt
1 cup brown rice crisp cereal

1. Line a small pan or container (about 4-by-4 inches) with parchment paper.
2. In a small saucepan, combine the honey, tahini, cinnamon, cardamom, and salt, and heat over low heat until the mixture is thin and smooth, about 1 minute.
3. Remove from the heat and stir in the brown rice crisp cereal, ensuring the mixture is cohesive.
4. Quickly place the mixture into the prepared pan and firmly press down, creating one even layer.
5. Refrigerate until firm and then slice into two large crispy rice treats.

VARIATION TIP: You can add chocolate chips, dried fruit, or even nuts and seeds to this recipe to make it your own.

Per serving: Calories: 216; Fat: 8g; Sodium: 171mg; Carbohydrates: 34g; Fiber: 1g; Sugar: 18g; Protein: 4g

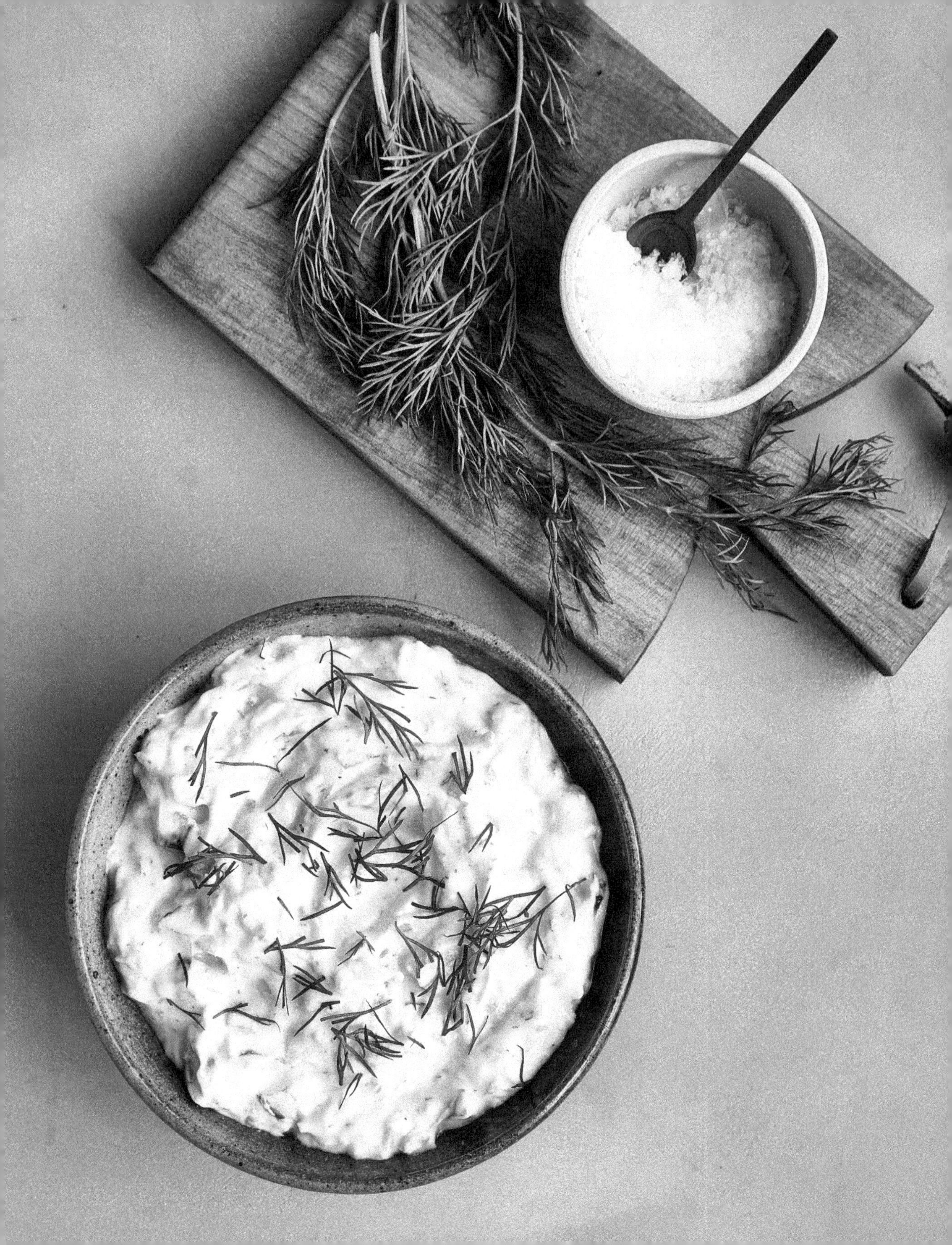

CHAPTER EIGHT

Staples

Spinach and Basil Pesto

Prep time: 5 minutes | Makes: 1½ cups

Quick, 5-Ingredient, One Pot, Gluten-Free, Vegetarian

Pesto is a great clean-eating staple to have on hand because you can blend it into sauces, drizzle it on sandwiches, use it as a dressing or marinade, and so much more. This pesto uses spinach, which increases the iron and magnesium content. Freeze pesto in ice cube trays for future use.

- 1 garlic clove, peeled
- 1 cup fresh basil
- 1 cup fresh baby spinach
- ½ cup grated Parmesan cheese
- 1 cup olive oil
- 2 teaspoons freshly squeezed lemon juice
- ½ teaspoon salt
- ¼ teaspoon freshly ground black pepper

In a food processor, lightly pulse the garlic. Add the basil, spinach, and Parmesan cheese, and pulse again to blend. Slowly drizzle the oil into the processor. Add the lemon juice, salt, and pepper, pulsing to combine.

VARIATION TIP: I like the blend of spinach and basil, but you can make this pesto with all basil or all spinach. Feel free to add walnuts or pine nuts, which are more traditional.

Per serving (1 tablespoon): Calories: 88; Fat: 9.5g; Sodium: 81mg; Carbohydrates: 0g; Fiber: 0g; Sugar: 0g; Protein: 0g

Everyday Salad Dressing

Prep time: 5 minutes | Makes: 1 cup

There's no need to purchase store-bought dressings when you can easily make your own at home. Wonderful on salads, this simple dressing is also great to drizzle on cooked fish or vegetables.

- ½ cup olive oil
- ⅓ cup freshly squeezed lemon juice
- 2 teaspoons maple syrup
- 1 teaspoon minced shallot
- ½ teaspoon salt
- ¼ teaspoon freshly ground black pepper
- 1 tablespoon chopped fresh parsley

In a resealable container or jar, combine the oil, lemon juice, maple syrup, shallot, salt, pepper, and parsley. Shake vigorously to mix well. Store in the refrigerator for up to 5 days.

VARIATION TIP: You can add many different spices, like basil or thyme, to this dressing.

SUBSTITUTION TIP: Try using different vinegars like red wine, champagne, or even plain white vinegar instead of the lemon juice for a more sour flavor.

Per serving (1 tablespoon): Calories: 63; Fat: 6.5g; Sodium: 73mg; Carbohydrates: 1g; Fiber: 0g; Sugar: 0.5g; Protein: 0g

Tahini Dressing

Prep time: 5 minutes | Makes: ¾ cup

Tahini is made from toasted sesame seeds, so it's a great source of protein, magnesium, and B vitamins. You can use this tahini dressing in the White Bean and Cilantro Hummus (page 101) instead of just tahini, or try drizzling it on top of the Chickpea Grain Bowls with Avocado and Feta (page 56).

- ¼ cup tahini
- ¼ cup olive oil
- 4 tablespoons water
- 2 teaspoons honey
- 1¼ teaspoons freshly squeezed lemon juice
- ¼ teaspoon ground cumin
- ¼ teaspoon ground cardamom

In a resealable container or jar, combine the tahini, oil, water, honey, lemon juice, cumin, and cardamon. Shake vigorously to mix well. Store in the refrigerator for up to 5 days.

COOKING TIP: If the dressing thickens up in the refrigerator, add 1 teaspoon of water at a time to loosen it up. Once opened, tahini can be stored in the refrigerator to help preserve the oils so they won't go rancid.

Per serving (1 tablespoon): Calories: 73; Fat: 7g; Sodium: 2mg; Carbohydrates: 2g; Fiber: 0g; Sugar: 1g; Protein: 1g

Quick, 5-Ingredient, One Pot, Dairy-Free, Gluten-Free, Vegetarian

Coconut Dressing with Honey and Lime

Prep time: 5 minutes | Makes: ½ cup

Quick, 5-Ingredient, One Pot, Gluten-Free, Vegetarian

This refreshing dressing tastes great on top of nearly any salad and is a nice, clean change from heavy, creamy dressings. The coconut milk is light and has a naturally sweet flavor. Try it as a dipping sauce with the Spiced Chicken Strips (page 92).

- ½ cup canned full-fat coconut milk
- 2 teaspoons plain low-fat yogurt
- 1 teaspoon honey
- 1 teaspoon freshly squeezed lime juice
- 1 teaspoon chopped chives
- ¼ teaspoon salt

In a resealable container or jar, combine the coconut milk, yogurt, honey, and lime juice. Mix well, then add the chives and salt. Stir to combine well. Store in the refrigerator for up to 5 days.

SUBSTITUTION TIP: If you don't have chives, try using scallions or shallots. Feel free to add parsley for more green color.

Per serving (1 tablespoon): Calories: 31; Fat: 3g; Sodium: 75mg; Carbohydrates: 1g; Fiber: 0g; Sugar: 0.5g; Protein: 0g

Vegetable Broth

Prep time: 5 minutes | Cook time: 30 minutes | Makes: 11 cups

One Pot, Gluten-Free, Vegan

Making your own is a great way to ensure your vegetable broth is high quality and nutrient dense. It's also a great way to use up some older vegetables or even vegetable scraps that you may have in your refrigerator. Once it's cooled, pack the broth in smaller containers and store in the freezer for later use.

- 7 celery stalks, cut into large pieces
- 1 onion, quartered
- 1 medium sweet potato, cut into 4 pieces
- 7 mushrooms, halved
- ½ bunch fresh parsley
- 2 bay leaves
- 2 thyme sprigs
- 2 teaspoons salt
- 1 teaspoon freshly ground black pepper

1. In a stock pot, combine the celery, onion, sweet potato, mushrooms, parsley, bay leaves, thyme sprigs, salt, and pepper. Fill with enough water to cover the vegetables and they begin to float.
2. Bring to a boil on high heat for 5 minutes. Then cover, reduce the heat to medium, and simmer for 25 minutes.
3. Strain the vegetables. Let the broth cool and store it in an airtight container in the refrigerator for up to 5 days or in the freezer for up to 6 months.

VARIATION TIP: The broth can be made with other vegetables, so feel free to use up what you already have in your refrigerator.

Per serving (1 cup): Calories: 5; Fat: 0g; Sodium: 441mg; Carbohydrates: 1g; Fiber: 0g; Sugar: 0.5g; Protein: 0g

Salsa

Prep time: 10 minutes | Makes: 6 cups

Quick, Gluten-Free, Vegan

Serve this refreshing dip with the Speedy Steak Fajitas (page 82) or as a finishing condiment on fish. It gives you so many nutrients, and there are no added preservatives or additives like in store-bought salsa.

- 6 plum tomatoes, cut into 6 chunks
- 1 large bunch cilantro, halved
- 1 green bell pepper, cut into 6 pieces
- 1 red bell pepper, cut into 6 pieces
- ½ sweet onion, quartered
- ½ medium red onion, quartered
- 1 medium jalapeño pepper, stemmed (seeds are optional)
- 1 garlic clove, peeled
- 1 cup low-sodium tomato juice
- Juice of 2 limes

1. In a food processor, pulse the tomatoes and cilantro until almost minced. Transfer to a bowl.
2. Add the bell peppers, sweet and red onions, jalapeño, and garlic to the food processor and pulse. Add the tomato juice and lime juice, then pour the tomatoes and cilantro back into the food processor and pulse until well blended.
3. Store in an airtight container in the refrigerator for up to 5 days or in the freezer for up to 3 months.

VARIATION TIP: You can use all red onion or eliminate the jalapeño pepper if you'd like. If you want just a little spice, add the jalapeño pepper but omit the seeds.

Per serving (¼ cup): Calories: 13; Fat: 0g; Sodium: 10mg; Carbohydrates: 3g; Fiber: 0.5g; Sugar: 1.5g; Protein: 0g

Strawberry Spread

Prep time: 5 minutes | Cook time: 30 minutes | Makes: 2 cups

Whether you are having a snack with afternoon tea or some whole-wheat toast for breakfast, this simple strawberry spread can make it a treat. It is low in sugar and has no preservatives. Strawberries are high in antioxidants, which help fight off inflammation.

---

2 cups frozen or fresh strawberries, trimmed and quartered
2 tablespoons honey
1 tablespoon water
1 tablespoon freshly squeezed lemon juice
1 teaspoon brown sugar
1 tablespoon chopped fresh mint

1. In a 2-quart pot, combine the strawberries, honey, and water over medium heat and stir constantly until the strawberries start to break down, 10 to 15 minutes. Add the lemon juice and brown sugar.
2. Using a potato masher, smash the strawberries. Reduce the heat to low and cook for about 15 minutes more, until the mixture starts to thicken. Add the mint during the last 5 minutes of cooking.
3. Store in an airtight container in the refrigerator for up to 2 weeks or in the freezer for up to 3 months.

COOKING TIP: Taste the berries beforehand to check for sweetness. Sometimes berries can be tart.

Per serving (1 tablespoon): Calories: 8; Fat: 0g; Sodium: 0mg; Carbohydrates: 2g; Fiber: 0g; Sugar: 1.5g; Protein: 0g

Carrot and Cucumber Yogurt Sauce

Prep time: 5 minutes | Makes: 1½ cups

Quick, 5-Ingredient, One Pot, Gluten-Free, Vegetarian

Easy to make and full of flavor, this yogurt sauce is great to have on hand. It pairs perfectly with the Ultimate Falafel Burgers (page 57) and can be served simply as a dip with some freshly sliced vegetables.

- 1½ cups plain low-fat Greek yogurt
- 6 tablespoons finely grated carrot
- 6 tablespoons diced cucumber
- 1 tablespoon freshly squeezed lemon juice
- ½ teaspoon dried dill
- Pinch salt
- Pinch freshly ground black pepper
- Chopped fresh dill, for garnish (optional)

1. In a resealable container or jar, combine the yogurt, carrot, cucumber, lemon juice, and dill, and mix well to combine. Season with the salt and pepper. Garnish with chopped fresh dill (if using).
2. Store in an airtight container in the refrigerator for up to 2 weeks.

VARIATION TIP: If you like garlic, try adding 1 minced garlic clove for even more flavor.

Per serving (¼ cup): Calories: 49; Fat: 1g; Sodium: 88mg; Carbohydrates: 4g; Fiber: 0g; Sugar: 2g; Protein: 6g

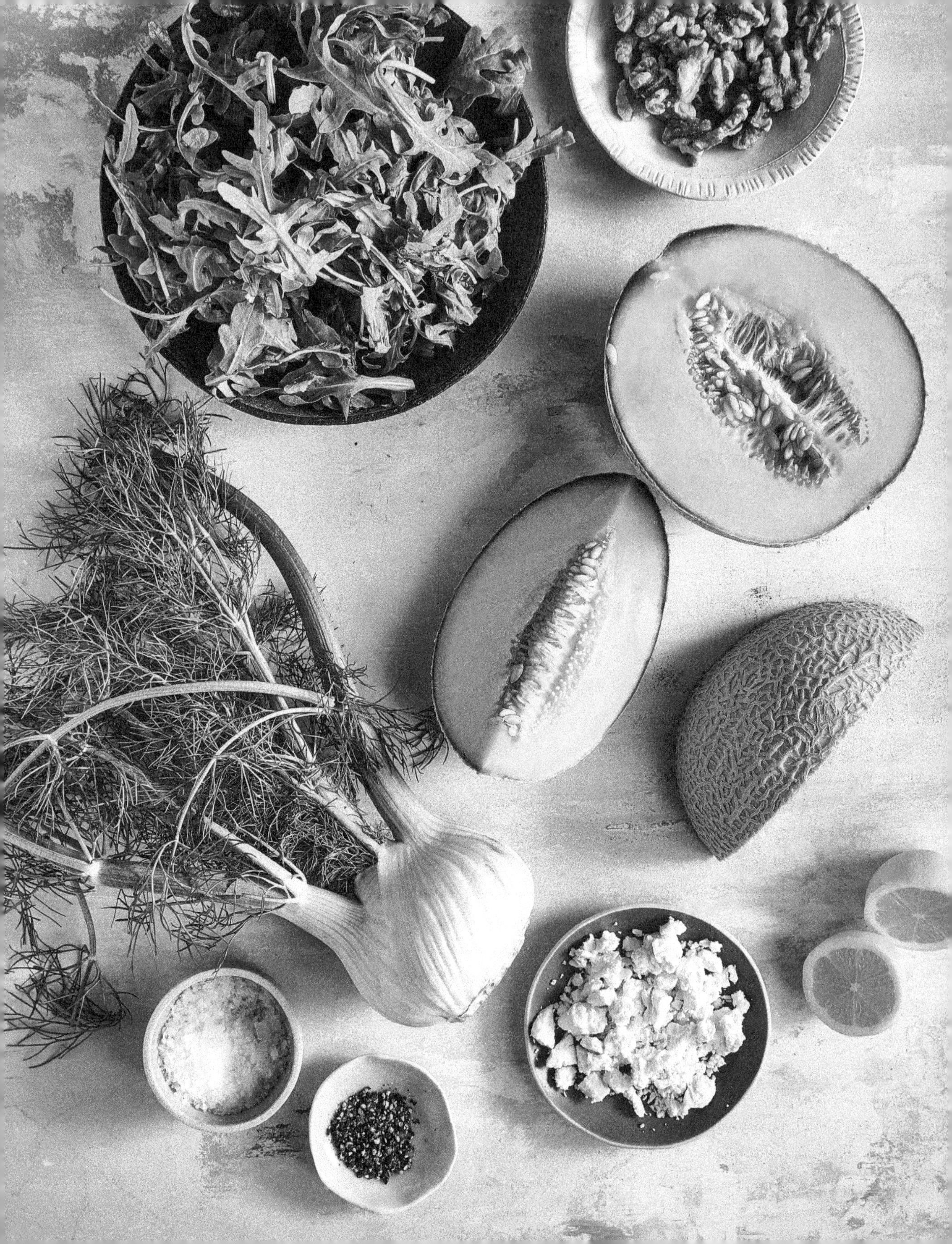

MEASUREMENT CONVERSIONS

	U.S. STANDARD	U.S. STANDARD (OUNCES)	METRIC (APPROXIMATE)
VOLUME EQUIVALENTS (LIQUID)	2 tablespoons	1 fl. oz.	30 mL
	¼ cup	2 fl. oz.	60 mL
	½ cup	4 fl. oz.	120 mL
	1 cup	8 fl. oz.	240 mL
	1½ cups	12 fl. oz.	355 mL
	2 cups or 1 pint	16 fl. oz.	475 mL
	4 cups or 1 quart	32 fl. oz.	1 L
	1 gallon	128 fl. oz.	4 L
VOLUME EQUIVALENTS (DRY)	⅛ teaspoon	———	0.5 mL
	¼ teaspoon	———	1 mL
	½ teaspoon	———	2 mL
	¾ teaspoon	———	4 mL
	1 teaspoon	———	5 mL
	1 tablespoon	———	15 mL
	¼ cup	———	59 mL
	⅓ cup	———	79 mL
	½ cup	———	118 mL
	⅔ cup	———	156 mL
	¾ cup	———	177 mL
	1 cup	———	235 mL
	2 cups or 1 pint	———	475 mL
	3 cups	———	700 mL
	4 cups or 1 quart	———	1 L
	½ gallon	———	2 L
	1 gallon	———	4 L
WEIGHT EQUIVALENTS	½ ounce	———	15 g
	1 ounce	———	30 g
	2 ounces	———	60 g
	4 ounces	———	115 g
	8 ounces	———	225 g
	12 ounces	———	340 g
	16 ounces or 1 pound	———	455 g

	FAHRENHEIT (F)	CELSIUS (C) (APPROXIMATE)
OVEN TEMPERATURES	250°F	120°C
	300°F	150°C
	325°F	180°C
	375°F	190°C
	400°F	200°C
	425°F	220°C
	450°F	230°C

INDEX

C

D

E

M

N

O

P

Q

R

S

T

U

V

W

Y

Z

ACKNOWLEDGMENTS

I want to thank many people for making this cookbook possible.

The first thank you goes to my husband, Eddie, who is always loving, supportive and proud of me, no matter what project I undertake. I thank my children, Caite and Brian, for enjoying food as much as I do and for your feedback and love throughout this process. You are the best taste testers I could ask for. Although my mother is deceased, she is here with me in spirit, and it's from her that I learned the beauty of scratch cooking nutritious, delicious meals. She also taught me by way of example the importance of nutritious food and the value of good health. Perhaps most important, she always taught me to reach for the stars.

I want to thank my sisters, Rita and Vera, and my brother-in-law Sean (my fellow foodie) for their wonderful, continuous support.

I cannot thank Erika Bay, my nutrition and dietetics intern, enough for her hard work, enthusiasm, and dedication. She kept me on track and in check at all times! Thank you, Christen Cooper, for your encouragement and believing in me. Thanks to all my friends for your feedback and support. I am proud and blessed to be surrounded by loving friends, family, and coworkers.

ABOUT THE AUTHOR

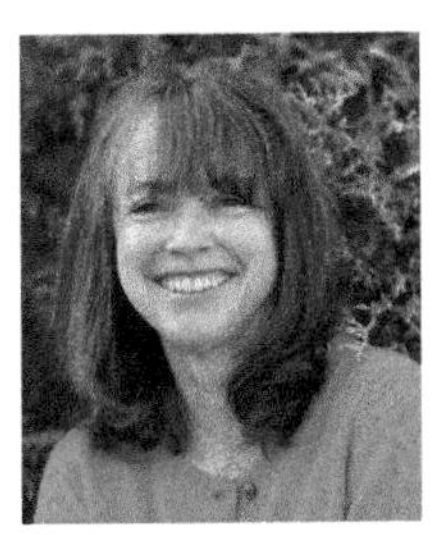

Mary Opfer is a registered dietitian nutritionist (RDN) with a master's degree from Teachers College, Columbia University, in New York. She is the founding clinical professor of culinary nutrition in the Master of Science in Nutrition and Dietetics Program at Pace University in Pleasantville, New York. She also maintains a private nutrition counseling practice, focusing on gastrointestinal and autoimmune disorders and weight loss.

Mary combined her career as a restaurateur with her scientific knowledge of food and cooking skills to develop numerous original recipes that appear in well-known cookbooks.

She has a passion for helping her community achieve better health through healthy cooking and has created a number of community-based meal planning and preparation classes. Mary is regularly quoted as a food and nutrition expert in national and international media outlets and has conducted nutrition webinars for a number of *Fortune* 500 companies.

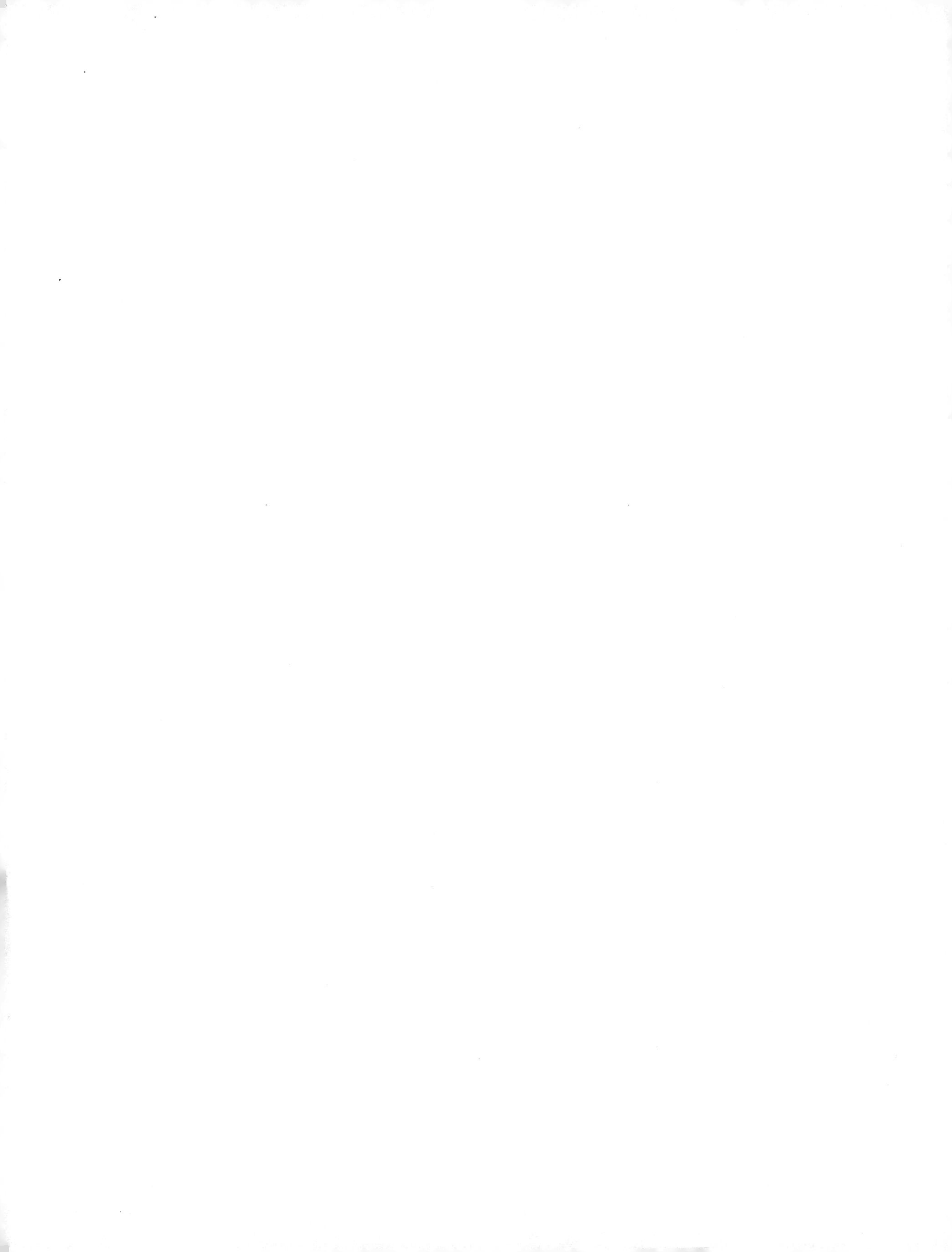

CPSIA information can be obtained
at www.ICGtesting.com
Printed in the USA
JSHW010259010821
17422JS00004B/8